P

ALZHEIMER
FOR FRIENDS AND RELATIVES

"After my diagnosis [with younger-onset Alzheimer's], many of my friends didn't know what to say to me. They thought, and some still do, that I couldn't think for myself, that I couldn't understand them, and they would talk around me, not to me. If I had had this book then, I would have given each one a copy and asked them to read it. As I read this book, my thoughts were—finally someone gets it and can make it easier on everyone."

— *Kris Bakowski, speaker and Alzheimer's advocate*

"Timely and concise, this essential book shows how to help a loved one with Alzheimer's disease or a caregiver on the frontlines. Brimming with compelling stories and practical advice, this guidebook will make an immediate and important difference in the lives of readers everywhere. As a survivor herself, Dr. Cail truly knows the subject and brings meaningful insight into the power of family and friends in hard times."

— *Ben Sherwood, President of ABC News, author of* The Survivors Club

"Mary Cail's book shows how to make friendships with Alzheimer's patients and their caregivers easy and rewarding, even during the late stage, which is so often hidden from the world. The book's epilogue is a game changer in terms of presuming to know with accuracy what perceptions fill the minds of patients who are unresponsive due to brain dysfunction or destruction by Alzheimer's disease. Friendship and even simple companionship are valuable at all stages of Alzheimer's disease."

— *Sam Gandy, M.D., Ph.D., Director of the Mount Sinai Center for Cognitive Health, Director of the NFL Neurological Center, Mount Sinai Chair in Alzheimer's Disease Research, Professor of Neurology and Psychiatry at Mount Sinai School of Medicine*

"Well written and compelling. An accurate portrayal for the person who wants to understand the experience of Alzheimer's disease from the perspective of both patient and carer."

— *Steven T. DeKosky, M.D., James Carroll Flippin Professor of Medical Science at the University of Virginia School of Medicine, recipient of the Rita Hayworth*

Award from the Alzheimer's Association, recipient of the Ronald and Nancy Reagan Institute Award, former Chair of the Alzheimer's Association Medical and Scientific Advisory Council

"An excellent, readable, fast-paced resource—unlike anything else on the market. I believe it will make a tremendous difference to people who must face this terrible disease."

—*Sue Friedman, President and CEO of the Alzheimer's Association, Central and Western Virginia*

"A sensitive and well-researched resource for 'all-weather friends' (caregivers, friends, family, or professionals)."

—*Cheryl Osborne, Ed.D., M.S.N., R.N., FAGHE, Director of Gerontology, Professor of Gerontology & Nursing, California State University Sacramento*

"An insightful, beautifully written guide that tells how to support and comfort friends dealing with Alzheimer's disease as either patients or caregivers. It provides a viable answer to the social isolation which so often becomes a part of dementia."

—*Ellen Phipps, coauthor of* Connections: Engagement in Life for Persons Diagnosed with Dementia

"As an academic physician with a clinical practice in family medicine, I see many patients who are affected by Alzheimer's disease. They often suffer from social isolation, frustration, and exhaustion, which are parts of this devastating condition physicians cannot directly treat. *Alzheimer's: A Crash Course for Friends and Relatives* is a compelling, easily readable book that skillfully addresses these problems, with accurate information and practical advice. It is a welcome addition to the care we can offer those directly affected, as well as a resource providing a more personal view to enlighten healthcare providers and others supporting this community."

—*Andrea M. Nazar, D.O., Professor of Clinical Science, West Virginia School of Osteopathic Medicine*

"A must read for the would-be good friend. Highly recommended."

—*Midwest Book Review*

Alzheimer's

A Crash Course
for Friends and Relatives

Mary McDaniel Cail, Ph.D.

True Wind
P R E S S

Chapel Hill, North Carolina

The present work appeared in an earlier version under the title *The All-Weather Friend's Guide to Alzheimer's Disease: Staying Connected to Loved Ones with Dementia and Their Caregivers.* ©2011 by Mary M. Cail.

Names and identifying characteristics of the individuals whose stories are told have been changed to protect privacy.

The All-Weather Friend and related logos and graphics are registered trademarks.

Truewind Press gratefully acknowledges permissions for quotations from Kris Bakowski, DaCapo Long Life (for Betsy Peterson), and David Wolpe.

Published by Truewind Press | info@truewindpress.com | www.truewindpress.com
Book design by Jon Marken, www.lamppostpublicity.com
Cover design by Mary Wagner
Printed in the United States of America

Publisher's Cataloging-in-Publication Data

Cail, Mary M.
    Alzheimer's : a crash course for friends and relatives / Mary McDaniel Cail ; [foreword by Barry Petersen].

    p. ; cm. — (The All-Weather Friend ; [1])

Previously published as: The all-weather friend's guide to Alzheimer's disease. 2011.
    Issued also as an ebook.
    Includes bibliographical references and index.
    ISBN-13: 978-0-9825751-2-3
    ISBN-10: 0-9825751-2-2

    1. Alzheimer's disease—Patients—Family relationships. 2. Alzheimer's disease—Patients—Care. 3. Friendship. 4. Caregivers. 5. Interpersonal relations. I. Petersen, Barry (Barry Rex), 1949- II. Title.

RC523.2 .C35 2013
362.196/831   2012954147

In loving memory of
Greg McDaniel, my brother.
Thank you for the feathers.

FOREWORD

My wife, Jan, was diagnosed with younger-onset Alzheimer's disease at age 55. Thus began a journey that was lonely, sad, exhausting, and physically dangerous to me as a caregiver.

This book has a lot to say about being a friend, both to caregivers and to dementia patients, at a time in life when friends are vital to survival. I have one supreme demand for any caregiver who is reading it: Survive.

Alzheimer's caregivers are usually selected not by training, but by geography. We are the closest person to the person with the disease. It could be a wife caring for her husband, or a daughter for a parent, or a brother for a sister. Caregivers often suffer depression that can spiral into even more serious health problems. Caregivers cope with endless, growing and sometimes irrational demands. One constant...as bad as it is today, it will almost surely get worse.

And here's the hardest part: Caregivers are alone. With almost any other disease, the person who is sick is part of the team. If someone you love is battling cancer, that person is part of the process, part of making decisions about their life, medicine, chemotherapy.

Not with Alzheimer's. If you are the caregiver holding this book, you're it. Doctors have few treatments and none that offer a cure or even slow the disease. The person with the disease will disappear ever more, making your struggle as a caregiver ever harder. It makes having friends who can begin to understand and listen with compassion all the more important.

If you're a friend or relative, seize the tools in this book. Learn the strategies. Read how others coped. Prepare for what is coming, but do so knowing that every Alzheimer's journey will be different.

And if you're a caregiver, most of all take care of you. You will be of no use to the person you are caring for if you are no longer here.

Survive. That will be your personal victory over this disease.

Emmy Award–winning journalist and author **Barry Petersen** *has been a CBS News Correspondent for more than three decades. He is the author of* Jan's Story: Love Lost to the Long Goodbye of Alzheimer's.

CONTENTS

Alzheimer's

*A Crash Course
for Friends and Relatives*

THE ALL-WEATHER FRIEND:
MARY'S STORY

"And yet the compensations of calamity are made apparent to the understanding also, after long intervals of time…a cruel disappointment, a loss of wealth, a loss of friends, seems at the moment unpaid loss, and unpayable. But the sure years reveal the deep remedial force that underlies all facts. The death of a dear friend, wife, brother, lover which seemed nothing but privation, somewhat late assumes the aspect of guide…."[1]

— RALPH WALDO EMERSON (1803-1882)

American essayist and philosopher who died unable to write his own name due to a progressive dementia, probably Alzheimer's disease

IT WAS EARLY EVENING IN FEBRUARY, twelve years ago. I should have been at home making spaghetti. Wayne and I always had spaghetti on Sunday nights. This was one of the rituals in our marriage, like the coffee shop on weekends and "I love you" as the last words said each day. The tomatoes were stewed and in the saucepan, onions chopped. A pot of salted water sat on a cold stove. I'd left the house to look for him, troubled by a vague, persistent worry.

An hour later, I had made my way around the almost vacant corridors of the hospital where he worked. I was crouched against a wall in the back wing, arms clasped around my head, screaming. He had taken his own life. I remember people in white coats running to his corner office, the best office—the one with a window. My screams were instinctive, dissociated from deliberateness or restraint. Someone, a nurse, I think, cupped her hands under my elbows, drew me to my feet, led me away. Still I screamed, unable to stop. I was conscious of the harsh sound echoing in the hallway, of the shadowless artificial light, and of my legs obediently walking. My body seemed dismembered, as though the instant I found him I had been torn apart. Finally the woman stepped in front of me and gave my shoulders a shake, saying, "Ma'am, ma'am! It's all right."

I was calm then. Eerily calm. The screams died within me as quickly as a blown match. I stared at her face, the perfectly drawn pink lipstick, the mascara clinging to her eyelashes. I was capable again of forming words, sickening and rational. "My husband is dead. It is not all right." Thus began an odyssey of grief that culminated in one of Emerson's compensations—a mission guided by the lessons of loss.

I WAS FORTY-TWO YEARS OLD. My family lived three hundred miles away. I worked as a writer in an upstairs room of our house with a cat for a companion. I was struggling with the emptiness of a recent miscarriage that happened after five years of infertility treatments. Wayne had been recovering from surgery for a brain tumor. This was my first experience with how profoundly brain health affects everything about life, even the will to live. He was suffering from vertigo, depressed, unable to think clearly or sleep. Frightened for him, I pulled away from my friends. I had no time or energy for anyone else. After his death, I felt deeply, irrevocably shattered. And I felt completely alone.

In the worst moments, the pain was so crushing I could not stand on my feet. I sank to my knees and wailed, beyond the relief even of tears. The mortgage and the pets, the bills and projects were no more than an assembly line of responsibilities to which I numbly attended. I relied on friends' inclusion of me in their family and everyday activities: dinner, a child's soccer game, a hike in the mountains—one truly awful play, set entirely in a graveyard. My life was a cobbling of snippets from other people's lives, bound by long stretches when I dealt with vise-like grief. I realized then how irreplaceable friends are in any situation that pushes a person to the margins.

I felt I had no viable future left; I wanted to die. This dark wish drew me to a nursing home where people crept along clutching the side rails of linoleum-tiled hallways and languished in wheelchairs parked in front of a television set. While friends my age continued with careers, carpooled children and took dancing lessons, I spent time with very old people, oddly comforted by the idea my own life would eventually end, probably in such a way. My next step was to the Alzheimer's Association, where I began to lead patient and caregiver support groups.

DURING THE INITIAL CATACLYSM OF LOSS, though, I made an appointment with a counselor, needing an outlet for my pent-up emotions. In her waiting room the first day, I cynically studied the decorating tricks meant to put people like me at ease: the muted colors, the fountain, the dish of water-smoothed pebbles. How could it really help, I wondered, to divulge my confidential mix of rage and sorrow to a stranger who'd do little more than murmur "I hear you" against the backdrop of a few framed diplomas. When she came for me, holding out a slender hand in greeting, I instantly shifted from the irrational notion that I had any exclusive rights to the experience of heartbreak. She was an attractive Candace Bergen type, wearing sensible khaki. She looked at me with one hazel eye. The other lid, stitched shut, sank into the hollow of an empty socket.

In a way, we are all like that counselor, dealing as best we can with our own limitations in perception. We can hardly untangle and lay out in accurate terms the force of emotion within ourselves, much less comprehend the innermost conflicts of another. However, this realization need not hinder the acts of kindness and companionship that are a lifeline for the person gripped in the undertow of an extraordinary hardship.

Some months from the night of my husband's death, I was horseback riding with a friend across a broad field with tones of ripened grain and sky muted in late August haze. Riding has been my solace since I was a leggy, awkward child and continues to be as the wrinkles of middle age settle into my face. She turned to me with a flash of unexpected tears and said, "I miss Wayne." We trotted on, our horses' hooves thudding rhythmically in the swaying grass. She took the reins in one hand every few seconds to wipe her eyes. I let my own tears spill, blown crazily from my cheeks by the hot breeze. Her gesture was small, but I still remember those moments of shared grief.

It took years for me to find my way back to a sense of peace and happiness. By living through one of life's fierce, sudden storms, I learned the value of sturdy relationships. Many face the onset of Alzheimer's disease as they grow older and are as removed from the mainstream as I was, as afraid of what the future might hold. In my support groups, the world seems divided between those whose lives are caught in the enviable whirl of normality and those whose lives are dictated by the needs of a spouse or parent, beset by the plagues of age, but no more capable of reasoning and self-control than a young child. Their justifiable lament? No one else understands.

While aware of this reality, I would add to it. No one understands completely. Empathy, however, can be learned. Most people don't know instinctively how to be comforting in the wake of an adversity they have not handled themselves. Those we love most, who have shared large parts of our lives, will not bear our same losses and struggles.

The All-Weather Friend as a concept came from my conviction that people mean well. They want to know how to help when their friends face a true calamity, rather than be fair-weather friends who fade into the background, uncertain about what to say and do. The best of our friends are made by this willingness to listen, risk, and connect when the rewards are intangible and not immediate. They're the friends who make life worth cherishing, even when it is painful and hard. I hope this book helps you to be an All-Weather Friend to a loved one with dementia or a caregiver—a friend who is convinced of the redemptive power in your efforts.

ABOUT THIS BOOK

Does someone you love have Alzheimer's disease (AD)? Is one of your friends, relatives, or neighbors a caregiver? You can make the most of your relationship from the early stage, when changes are not so obvious, through the last. If a person in your world is dealing with AD, whether as a patient or a caregiver, this book is for you. It will guide you through steps you can take to be sensitive and supportive in the months and years ahead. You can help more than you may believe possible just by learning new ways to connect.

The book can best be described as a crash course for people who have not experienced this situation themselves. In a crash course, information is practical, often used to tackle a crisis. It breaks the surface and invites a more in-depth investigation. Most of us, however, are quite familiar with Alzheimer's disease, given the intense media coverage of late. We don't want so many details. The neurobiology is thoroughly complicated. What we can readily see—the relentless loss of intellect and life skills—is grim.

A man I met at a party was more candid than most when I told him I was writing about friendship and dementia. He paused for a moment and asked, smiling politely, "Why would I want to read that?" as if to say, Why would anyone? His hesitation was not surprising. An affliction that slips in and stealthily destroys neurons frightens us. We are tempted to push the threat to the fringes of conscious thought, eat salmon and blueberries (linked to a lowered risk of cognitive decline), and hope for the best. We abandon, sometimes, the people who must squarely face the disease.

But the single biggest risk factor for AD is age. By placing ourselves well within the orbit of modern medicine and complying with the roster of recommended health screenings, most of us try earnestly to become old. Ironically, our success in prolonging life is related to the disease's prevalence. In the year 2050, one in eight people worldwide will be over the age of sixty-five. At present, one in eight people over sixty-five has Alzheimer's disease. The longer you live, the greater the chance Alzheimer's will affect your life in a significant way, if it hasn't already.

THIS BOOK IS MEANT TO HELP YOU navigate the changes AD brings to friendships with dementia patients and their caregivers. The book is organized into four independent parts, beginning with essential background information. While reading about plaques and tangles may seem less important than the "how to" material which follows, learning the facts of a friend's condition is a kindness he or she will most certainly appreciate. The effort to bring others up to speed about a problem can add to the stress: It is exhausting to repeat the same information over and over, even when you are grateful for people's interest and concern.

The effort to bring others up to speed about a problem can add to the stress: It is exhausting to repeat the same information over and over, even when you are grateful for people's interest and concern.

The first three parts are about life with the disease after it has passed the preclinical (or asymptomatic) stage, in which changes are occurring in the brain, but outward signs are not yet evident.* Stories are followed by suggestions that explain how to support both the friend with memory loss and the caregiver.

Part Four opens with the story of a book publisher, Bert Brown, and his wife, Willa, a physician who began to have problems with short term memory at the height of her career in national public health. Willa quickly lost her ability to think coherently, but Bert's devotion to her

---

*For clarification, the first three parts of this book correspond to the seven stages you'll find listed on the Alzheimer's Association website (www.alz.org) as follows: *Mild Decline*, stages three and four; *Mid-Stage*, five and six; *The Last Years*, stage seven.

remained steady. While giving a snapshot of the isolation any type of dementia can bring about, it is also a love story—an example of the enduring, unconditional love we crave in this inconstant world but seldom find. Chapter 11, *Seven Ways to Stay Connected*, gives methods of reaching out as dementia becomes more demanding and alienating. Chapter 12 describes a dinner party attended by a seventy-five-year old woman with advanced AD and her husband, then her caregiver. None of the other guests had met her ahead of time. As the chapter shows, given consideration, some people with dementia can both enjoy and participate in such a gathering. The ending, almost unbelievably, is also a true story, hopefully an uplifting one, which makes a case for the possibility of an awareness untouched by dementia, close to the end, when everything appears to be lost.

Keep in mind, although the focus is on Alzheimer's, there are many other causes of dementia, and the resulting needs are much the same. For the purposes of this book, the terms are almost interchangeable.[2] Realize, too, that every person's experience of Alzheimer's disease is different. Medical science may be methodical and precise; relationships are more of a constantly evolving, creative art. The tips and strategies are meant to serve as guidelines. Do the best you can. A caregiver whose husband in mid-stage AD tends to sit for long stretches, disconcertingly silent and somber, has this advice: "People fear his lack of a response. They feel responsible and afraid if it doesn't go well. I want to say to them, 'Don't be afraid. It isn't your fault. I know he enjoys your company, even if he can't show it. And it means a lot to me when you spend time with him.'"

> *"People fear his lack of a response. They feel responsible and afraid if it doesn't go well. I want to say to them, 'Don't be afraid. It isn't your fault.'"*

YOU CAN MAKE A UNIQUE CONTRIBUTION to the lives of dementia patients and their caregivers. You understand the history—the important people, events, and places—upon which your relationship is based. You can reminisce with a friend suffering from Alzheimer's, and you can relate meaningfully to the broader circumstances of the caregiver's life. As someone who does not directly bear the problems and challenges, but can come and go at will, you may bring a different strength and energy to the situation.

We choose friends initially out of a sense of mutual benefit and enjoyment, avoiding, as a rule, people who talk too much or too little, people with overwhelming needs, and people with whom we do not share common interests and activities. However, we remain involved with friends caught up in trouble who may, in their struggles, temporarily show these same characteristics because we care about them: They've become a part of our lives; the relationship has deepened. When Alzheimer's affects the way a person can respond within a relationship or the way a caregiver can participate, the concept of reciprocity must be redefined. We stay connected as an expression of commitment and generosity. During the most difficult points of life, every person needs the unselfish attention of friends and loved ones who are willing to put aside some of their own needs and allow the relationship to adapt to the changing circumstances.

If you want to be a well-prepared All-Weather Friend, ready to view the gathering clouds of dementia as a reason to stick around rather than run for cover, then read on. Whether you have a lot of time or a little, you will make a difference.

ALZHEIMER'S 101

Sometimes she greets the doctor as if he were a visitor and excuses herself that she has not finished her work; on other occasions, she screams that he wants to cut her open; on others, she dismisses him, full of indignation and with expressions indicating that she fears him as a threat to her honor as a woman. At times, she is totally delirious.... Often, she screams for many hours in a horrible voice.[3]

— ALOIS ALZHEIMER, 1907

A HUNDRED YEARS AGO, a German railway clerk whose days were likely spent doling out tickets to a steady course of strangers became a stranger in his own home. Karl Deter's work may have been a monotonous grind of paper pushing, but his nightlife was shocking. His wife, Auguste, although unable to remember his name, shrieked accusations of infidelity at him. She insisted he was sleeping with the next-door neighbor; she despaired that the woman wanted to kill her. She dragged her bed linens around the house in the middle of the night in agitation and fell into long inconsolable tantrums.[4] One can imagine Deter, plodding home in his stiff dark uniform, trying in vain to apply the same logic to his wife that served him well in the predictable train station. The poor man must have wanted to flee to the arms of the next-door neighbor. In desperation he took Auguste to the family doctor, who wrote a prescription for her admission to the Hospital for the Mentally Ill and Epileptics in Frankfurt. Her physician at the institution was Alois Alzheimer.

By the early 1900s, care of the mentally ill had moved beyond the cruelties of the previous century. Patients were not bled, immobilized on tranquilizer chairs, spun in circles until dizzy, or used as a form of public entertainment. Nonetheless, they were subjected to weird physical indignities aimed, it seems, more at ensuring quietness and submission than treating the condition at hand. Auguste entered the asylum during the era of hydrotherapy, which involved wrapping patients in wet sheets or placing them in baths or showers, sometimes for longer than a day. Hydrotherapy was at the cutting edge of psychiatry, along with Freud's theory of memory loss as an indication of repressed trauma.

A physician had nothing more sophisticated to rely on for making a diagnosis than a microscope. The better part of a century would pass before the invention of medical scanners able to measure tissue volumes and metabolism in different regions of the brain. Until recently physicians could not examine living brain tissue in sufficient detail to make a definitive diagnosis without drilling into the skull for a biopsy, which is considered too invasive and risky. With the technology and combinations of methods now available, the clinical diagnosis is almost always accurate. Due to the slight uncertainty, patients are told they have *possible* or *probable* Alzheimer's disease.[5]

Alzheimer asked his patient simple questions.

"What is your name?"

"Auguste."

"Last name?"

"Auguste."

"What is your husband's name?"

"Auguste, I think."

"On what street do you live?"

"I can tell you. I must wait a bit." [6]

What color is snow? Soot? The sky? How many fingers do you have? Within a short time, Alzheimer corroborated the family doctor's report. Auguste was suffering from what he termed "a general imbecility" that failed to fit the pattern of any then classified disease. Her face was creased with distress and her eyes shadowed in weary circles, yet she had the long black hair and strong hands of her youth. Auguste was fifty-one years old, and her dementia had surfaced over the brief period of eight months. Alzheimer was mystified.

ALMOST FIVE YEARS LATER, lying in a fetal curl, Auguste died of sepsis from an infected bedsore. Alzheimer, who had moved on to the Royal Psychiatric Clinic in Munich, had her brain and medical records sent to him by train, possibly a train exiting the station where Auguste's husband still thumbed through schedules and fares, counted out change, and perhaps returned home evenings to a peaceful but lonely kitchen—made less lonely a year after his wife's death by his marriage to the neighbor she feared.[7] Alzheimer used his microscope and a new method of staining cells to study her neuroanatomy in painstaking detail.

In about a third of the neurons in Auguste's cerebral cortex, he saw thickened tangles of the threadlike filaments that normally run the length of the cell. In healthy neuronal cells, tau, a type of protein, binds these filaments so they can convey nutrients and other life sustaining material. In sketches Alzheimer made in his notebook, they look more like webs of knotted string than well-traveled cellular supply routes. The cause appears to be a molecular imbalance. Think of an eighteen-wheeler crossing a country bridge built to carry no more than the weight of a pickup truck. Under this burden, the protein disengages, and the microtubules collapse and fold within the cell, which is then no longer viable.

Alzheimer also saw numerous clumps of "a pathological metabolic product," which resembled birdseed, stuck together in dark globs and strewn throughout the outer layers of her brain. He used the word *miliary* (like millet seeds) to describe the deposits. Apparently at a loss for scientific nomenclature, he called these simply "a peculiar substance." Plaques, like tangles, are largely made up of a protein gone awry. The protein in its parent form, amyloid precursor protein or APP, is manufactured within neurons and other cells throughout the body. APP is processed by enzymes into derivative proteins, some of which may help to regulate and maintain synapses, the electronic pathways neurons use to communicate with one another by means of neurotransmitters. Neurotransmitters collectively make up a chemical pony express that rapidly dispatches messages across the synaptic spaces existing between each neuron in the human brain.

In Alzheimer's disease, maladaptive enzymes, acting like scissors in the hands of a poorly trained seamstress, snip off fragments of APP as the newly formed protein extrudes from the neuron. The result is a sticky amyloid-beta peptide, abnormal in structure and apparently toxic to the brain. These peptides accumulate around synapses and clump along with disintegrating nerve and inflammatory cells into the plaques Alzheimer described as scattered throughout Auguste's cortex.[8]

Alzheimer revealed his findings at a professional conference and summarized the presentation in a two-page abstract written clearly enough to be understood by a smart high school student. A century later, while we know more about the biology and genetics of Alzheimer's disease, medical science cannot give much in the way of lasting practical help to the twenty-six to thirty million people worldwide who, like Auguste Deter, are losing their minds, some much more quickly than others.

Considerable research has been focused, often with conflicting results, on detecting factors that may influence the emergence of full-fledged Alzheimer's disease.

Considerable research has been focused, often with conflicting results, on detecting factors that may influence the emergence of full-fledged Alzheimer's disease. The brains of some asymptomatic elderly people show evidence of the hallmark plaques of AD, yet these people have no appreciable mental decline as they grow older. A percentage of the cases of younger-onset AD, diagnosed before age sixty-five, are caused by a mutation in an autosomal dominant gene, meaning the child of a parent with the disease has a fifty percent chance of inheriting it. If so, she will become ill sometime after the age of thirty and well before retirement. Many of the geographically far flung families plagued by a high incidence of this rare variant can trace their ancestry to a group of Germans who migrated to Russia in the 1700s and lived in one of two villages flanked by the Volga River.

Others who develop AD have a genetic predisposition that interacts with environmental components to usher in dementia at a later age.[9] This setup is less a direct order than a strong suggestion. If you've inherited a tendency, for instance, toward high cholesterol, you may be more at risk for heart disease than someone else. Spend a lot of time sitting behind a desk with your susceptibility genes, smoking and eating fast food lunches, and you increase the odds these genes will eventually demand a spotlight on center stage, probably in the form of bypass surgery. But a healthy lifestyle does not assure protection against the dysfunctional players in your genetic profile, as conversely, a terrific set of genes is no guarantee of a life free from chronic disease. With thousands of genes constituting the chromosomes of cells in the human body, it is too complex an arrangement to allow for an unerring interpretation.

Alzheimer's disease percolates at a subclinical level for a decade or more, quietly obliterating neurons in and around the hippocampus, a paired structure deep in the right and left temporal lobes of the brain. The hippocampus is vital to forming new memories and maintaining proper orientation in space and time. Although the cellular changes that lead to the most common form of AD can begin in one's forties or earlier, this loss may not be noticed until it is widespread enough to cause obvious impairment. Delaying the disease's foray into conscious experience—problems with word retrieval, spatial relationships, time, initiative, and short-term memory—would, for many people, effectively prevent it: They would die before their brains degenerated in devastating measure.

ALZHEIMER'S DISEASE HAS NO CURE AT PRESENT. A list of foods, supplements, and circumstances which could interact with one's genetic blueprint to postpone or maybe prevent cognitive decline has sprung from experiments with genetically altered mice and controlled observations of people. Additions and revisions to the list trickle steadily into the lay press, but slowing AD may be like riding a horse. You can haul back on the reins with antioxidants, omega fatty acids, curcumin, aerobic exercise, and other tactics to little effect if the horse is already galloping at top speed. If the horse has just ambled out of the barn, health conscious habits established early on might have a positive impact on cognitive ability in the long run. Disturbingly though, the disease can gain a stronghold in the brain regardless of any efforts to thwart it.

Treatments cannot prevent or undo plaques and tangles. They can help with symptoms, like depression and agitation, or enable a person to carry out ordinary tasks for a while longer than would be possible otherwise. Medications will not restore memory, reverse damage already done to the brain, or arrest the disease. The medications at hand do not work for everyone and, when effective, result in limited improvements. This underwhelming response to treatment may be due to the fact much change within the brain has already occurred, hence the effort among scientists to find ways of suppressing the disease before the onset of dementia.

For the most part, drugs now on pharmacy shelves are intended to prevent the breakdown of acetylcholine, a neurotransmitter that becomes depleted as plaques increase, or to enhance neurotransmitter function in other ways. Think of fighting a fire by temporarily shoring up a flagging bucket brigade instead of shooting streams of water at the flames. A new generation of drugs under study in clinical trials is expected to inhibit or clear amyloid-beta accumulation in the brain. Some scientists believe this alternative will aim more directly at the fire. [10]

The sequence of losses caused by Alzheimer's disease and the approximate duration of its stages can be compared to a reverse of the developmental milestones from infancy to adulthood.[11] Psychiatrist Barry Reisberg mapped the system of changes, upon which the Alzheimer's Association now bases its seven-stage framework, and introduced the term "retrogenesis" to identify the process. A person with mild Alzheimer's disease has the competencies of an eight- to twelve-year-old: She can dress herself properly and keep track of uncomplicated finances. By mid-stage, this wrinkled and gray haired person is more like a very young child, without the endearing future promise and convenient small size. She cannot be left unsupervised; she may not remember how to open a can of soup, heat it, or use a spoon to feed herself. Finally, unless death comes prematurely from another cause, she will be unable to lift her head and, like a newborn, she will need constant care.

The fetal brain, however, develops neurons at a rate of 250,000 per minute from the first month of conception. The downy cheeked infant who can hardly do more than cry and sleep has one hundred billion of the cells, ready to respond at warp speed to the effects of physical maturation, sensory input, and experience. One can infer from those numbers how many neurons must be effaced by AD at a steady rate to return a person decades old, with a brain crammed full of information, to a state of profound helplessness, lacking in the end even an infant's impulse to swallow.

IN THE WAKE OF PUBLICITY about the relationship between aging and Alzheimer's disease,[12] the seventy-eight million baby boomers who are slipping, as Ronald Reagan put it, into their sunset years have become more circumspect about senior moments. We find it alarming to extrapolate from the occasional hitch in memory to a complete inability to think and function, and confronted by someone else's plight, tend to take refuge in the self-protective if blindly optimistic adage "This won't happen to me." Given the prevalence of Alzheimer's disease, it could happen to any of us. And we'd be caught up, then, in the terrible uncertainty of whether medical advances will be made soon enough for our benefit. Scientists may not be able to rout out a process lodged at the molecular level in the most sophisticated piece of anatomical engineering in existence. Although researchers are steadily uncovering genetic factors, developing methods of early identification, and exploring new treatments (some intended for the very earliest stage of the disease), hope of a cure in the near future is unrealistic.

Think of how you would feel, sitting across the desk from a neurologist as he or she confirmed your own diagnosis of Alzheimer's.* You'd want the reassurance loved ones and friends would stand by both you and your caregiver. If you wonder how you can help someone already on the difficult path of losing control of what she has spent a lifetime becoming or watching this happen to a person she loves, the chapters which follow will provide the ideas and strategies you need, as well as help you to understand the problems of living with this disease.

---

* In medical literature, the apostrophe is sometimes omitted ("Alzheimer disease"). The trend may be moving gradually away from use of the possessive for eponyms, but it remains the prevalent form in most nonmedical environments.

PART ONE

Mild Decline

1

Adelle's Story

I don't golf much anymore. I have arthritis in my hand, so it doesn't bother me not to be able to golf. There are about twelve of us who have a putting group at the country club. We putt, and then we have lunch. I can't always follow the conversation, but I like to sit and enjoy the company. I frankly think I've done very well to have had this disease for as long as I have. I'm careful about what I do. I get frustrated if I think of something and then can't remember how to say it. I realize it may be normal forgetting, but because I have this disease, I blame it on that.

— ADELLE, *diagnosed with Alzheimer's disease in 2001 at age 77*

WITH HER REFINED VOICE AND MANNER, Adelle might have had a privileged upbringing. She has the natural reserve that often accompanies wealth, but in fact, she and her brother spent much of their childhood abandoned at a boarding house in Detroit. The landlady was a single woman with a kind heart; she saved Adelle. She saw that two children were alone upstairs without enough food and discreetly became their

19

surrogate mother. She would pull Adelle onto her lap and reassure her of love and any security she could provide. "Those are moments I'll never forget my whole life," Adelle told one of her daughters, more than seventy years later.

She didn't talk to her own children about her past until they were older. To the children, "Grandma" was an infrequent visitor, not an alcoholic who had used their mother as a commodity. When she lived for erratic periods at the boarding house, Adelle's mother hired her young daughter out to clean house for bar cronies and pocketed the profits. Adelle remembers standing beside her brother on city sidewalks in winter with her bare feet wrapped in newspaper, selling apples for two cents each. Those times seem far removed from her current life in Naples, Florida. Nine years into a diagnosis with AD, she still drives herself to a salon for pedicures. She sometimes falls asleep in the chair now and tosses her credit card on the counter with no real thought of the bill. Her husband, Gary, carefully monitors the charges.

Adelle's early life was a mystery before her oldest daughter, Nancy, became her part-time caregiver. Since the diagnosis, Nancy has commuted several hundred miles to the home of her mother and stepfather, staying with them for weeks at a time. Gary, in his early eighties, runs his own company. Adelle can no longer serve as his bookkeeper, and the hours alone while he works at the office would be tedious for her. Nancy and her mother pal around together, shopping at the mall, having lunch, and reading. Nancy describes their relationship as stronger and more intimate. "I've developed a closeness with my mother I didn't have before," she says. "I've gotten to know her as adult woman to adult woman. This has been able to happen even with the Alzheimer's, because most of the time you don't notice that she has it. She can be wise and insightful. She just repeats herself a lot. We talk for hours, and she tells me things from her childhood I've never heard before."

Adelle could have been embittered by her early years, spent in such poverty that she was never allowed the luxury of a toothbrush. Against all odds, she grew into an easygoing young woman, quick to laugh, and gifted with an unusually dazzling smile. Nancy thought of her as the mother who could do anything. The only time she saw Adelle on a minor rampage was when her younger sister, Stella, returned home from the beauty shop on the night of her prom. Stella burst through the door in tears, with a hairpiece that looked like a bird's nest teased into the top of her head. "Get in the car!" Adelle ordered and drove her back to the salon. To Stella's shock, she stormed in and cornered the hapless beautician. "Would *you* want your hair done like this?!" she demanded. The mistake was remedied, and Adelle returned to her unflappable demeanor. She seldom again showed such agitation until Alzheimer's disease began to erode her capacity for self-control.

Adelle fully cares for herself. She dresses meticulously, though sometimes in the same outfit on consecutive days, forgetting she has worn it already. For the most part, time goes gently along, and the disease is more a great inconvenience than a disabling handicap. The symptoms overtake her, though, with a vengeance at unpredictable intervals. In the mall one morning, she suddenly became terrified of the escalator. "She stood at the bottom," Nancy remembers, "and started screaming, 'No! No! No!! I can't do it! I can't do it!' I ran back down the stairs and said, 'It's okay. You don't have to! We'll take the elevator.' Then she was fine. Everything was back to normal."

IN EARLY ALZHEIMER'S, "NORMAL" is no longer the usual state, in which there is hardly an awareness of the brain because it does the job as always, like an efficient administrator in a plain gray suit. Thirty-year-olds are not concerned when they mislay the cell phone or forget why they have gone upstairs. Absentmindedness from time to time is part of the human condition. As the disease whittles away the hippocampus, this reliance on the brain's stability shifts to preoccupation with its more frequent failures. The amused expression, "Sorry, I had a senior moment!" turns into "My God, what is happening to me?" asked in genuine fear.

The process can occur so insidiously a person passes from the early into the mid-stage without being conscious of the change.[13] But for many, the early stage is as menacing as a gathering war on home soil. A caregiver, Ethel, walked into the kitchen one day and found her husband sitting at the table with his head in his hands. "I'm losing it," he said and began to cry. His mother was in the late stage of the disease at the time and lived in their home. Ethel, a petite woman with her own inventory of health problems, eventually had to care for both of them.

Alzheimer's disease is strangely deniable even to family and friends witnessing the overt evidence of it in someone they love. The first indications are so benign and commonplace: a forgotten appointment here and there, a lost name or train of thought, an overdrawn bank account.

The disease is strangely deniable even to family and friends.

Haven't most of us blundered in these areas? I regularly misplace my reading glasses. I've tied my house keys to my wallet with a ribbon. I rely heavily on my desk calendar to keep track of appointments. At some point, a slow descent into discernible dementia becomes unmistakable, but acceptance of the condition is often dragged into a long saga that in hindsight can seem almost ludicrous. Virginia, a college professor whose husband, Andrew, is a Harvard-educated physician, said he once left their daughter's house for a walk and didn't return. After a few hours, Virginia frantically called the police. They found him several doors down, curled up asleep on a neighbor's couch, and brought him home unscathed. "Hmm, it is odd," she and her son (also a physician) agreed, musing in relief. "But, you know, he never did pay much attention to the interior decorating."

Adelle's diagnosis capped a two-year period in which problems became increasingly evident to her family, despite her attempts to hide them. "Don't you remember telling me that?" Stella would ask, when her mother repeated herself. Adelle replied reassuringly that she was only making sure Stella had heard her. The point of no return in the family's collective worries happened on Thanksgiving. Adelle was an accomplished cook who had presided through the years like an army general over holiday dinner preparations. That fateful day, as her daughters and husband scurried in her wake, she absentmindedly picked up a pan of soapsuds and poured it into the gravy.

Until then, they had accepted the family doctor's opinion of her memory lapses. He dismissed the concern in hand and so did a psychiatrist, called upon for a second opinion. Finally a neurologist made the diagnosis after the customary battery of tests, in which an MRI showed the telltale pattern of brain atrophy associated with AD. Gary shifted into high gear, determined to leave no stone unturned in finding help for his wife. He heard about patient selection for the clinical trial of AN-1792, the Alzheimer's vaccine developed by the Dublin-based drug company, Elan, and managed, through a barrage of email messages, faxes and phone calls, to secure one of the coveted places in the study for Adelle. She was to receive six injections that would prompt her own immune system to attack the amyloid-beta in her brain. After she began the treatment, Gary noticed an almost immediate leveling out of her memory problems, and his hopes ran high. In mid-January of 2002, they arrived at the hospital for the third injection but were turned away at the door. The trial had been halted by an urgent message received only minutes earlier, when investigators confirmed brain inflammation in a small percentage of the almost four hundred study participants. No amount of persuasion could change the decision. In a last-ditch bid, Gary called executives at Elan and offered to take Adelle to the company's headquarters in Ireland to continue the treatment.

Afterward they found themselves in the same boat as everyone else, making use of the drugs currently available for treatment and making plans for the future. Adelle's reaction to the diagnosis had been typical. She thought it was a death sentence. "I'm no good to anybody," she sometimes laments during periods of depression. "They ought to take me out back and shoot me." Gary set the stage for accepting with dignity what they could not change. They didn't conceal her condition from friends, nor did they withdraw socially. There was never any shame. Knowledge of the disease was a new reality to be faced and accommodated.

The family inadvertently looked to Gary for how to handle Adelle's problems with memory and her uncharacteristic outbursts of temper, and he has provided an example of unfailing patience. He consistently responds to her as though hearing for the first time the things she repeats—on bad days, over and over. "Gary, have you seen my purse?" she might ask. *It's right beside you, Adelle.* "Gary, have you seen my purse?" she'll say again, five minutes later. *It's right beside you, Adelle.* "Gary, I can't find my purse!" *It's right beside you, Adelle.* He doesn't change his tone or facial expression. If she asks the same question ten times, he answers ten times without a hint of aggravation. He has given her the gift of being able to live with her disease unburdened by the worry of his frustrations. As a result, Adelle does not have a sense of how forgetful she really is. The brain without a hippocampus, a dated analogy goes, is like a tape recorder running with no tape. Everything seems to be in working order. The batteries are fresh, the gears are turning, but nothing, once the hippocampus is finally gone, can be stored. Gary realizes how hurt Adelle would be if he reacted to her repetitiousness with exasperation, no matter how forgivable. He knows she cannot help herself and keeps this thought planted firmly in the front of his mind.

Gary's effort to protect Adelle from the emotional pain of her mental decline may lack the stage worthiness of a movie romance, but it is nonetheless a dramatic example of love and humanity. He met Adelle when she was in her early fifties, ten years after Nancy and Stella's young father died of a heart attack. Despite this tragedy and her long final struggle with AD, she is a woman who would be envied by many of her peers. Two devoted men have successively shared most of her adult life, and although she cannot remember anything from one minute to the next, she describes herself as a happy person. No great wonder. Happiness and love have long been linked. "I'm content," she says. "I have what I need. Gary is a very positive person, and I do whatever I can to keep my mind active."

This is not to paint too rosy a picture. Alzheimer's disease exponentially increases the difficulty of virtually every situation. A gall bladder operation she underwent several years ago turned into a nightmare for everyone involved. Her husband and children stood outside a hospital room, listening in sick helplessness to her shrieks of panic through the walls. "No! Nooo! Don't do it! *Don't!*" she screamed in childlike terror, as physicians performed invasive tests and treatments. At least, Nancy later commented, they realized Adelle would have no lasting memory of it.

On another occasion, the family colluded to keep a secret from one member to protect the privacy of another. They had carefully worked out the details of how this would be accomplished, and everything went along swimmingly until Adelle, who had forgotten, innocently blurted out the truth. "Oh, no!" she agonized in the aftermath. "Oh, no. I am so stupid. How stupid, stupid, stupid! Oh, I'm so stupid." Early AD is capricious—one fact of the recent past is forgotten and another remembered with less reliability than penny stocks. The precise alliances between neurons responsible for encoding new memories no longer exist. To illustrate, think how different the outcome would have been for the United States at the 1992 Olympics if players on the Dream Team had jogged off the basketball court from time to time without warning. Thus Adelle could hold the memory of her mistake long enough to fall into a forty-five minute fit of self-recrimination for having forgotten her role in the family crisis when it really mattered.

> *Early AD is capricious—one fact of the recent past is forgotten and another remembered with less reliability than penny stocks.*

Robert, a psychiatrist in the early stage of AD, can remember, almost chillingly, having lost a pair of shoes and the details of his scramble to reason where they were. "Even in the midst of this disease, I try to apply an Aristotelian logic, but it's confused," he explained. "I couldn't find the shoes and thought, 'Oh, I was at my daughter's house last night. That's it! I went up to her bedroom and took a nap. I must have taken them off beside the bed.' It didn't occur to me how impossible it would have been to leave her house that night in my socks. You come to these conclusions that are crazy and distorted." In his clear-thinking recollections of these incidents, Robert shows the huge reserves of intellect that remain in early AD, not so much what has been stripped away. "It's like living in a dream in which things don't fit together," he said, trying to find words that would convey the experience. "I feel distanced from everyone, somehow not involved in the world anymore."

Twenty years older than Robert, Adelle stays within the boundaries of her family and circle of closest friends and doesn't feel the same sting of isolation. With the passing of time, her loved ones have adjusted as necessary to the changes. At first, it was hard not to look ahead and despair over what would happen to her in unrelenting increments. Stella, genetically endowed with her mother's smile and probably a certain indomitable optimism, adopted a "glass half full" attitude. "Let's not worry about tomorrow," she counseled. "Let's enjoy her while we can. Tomorrow may never come."

They have learned to categorically ignore disease-driven behaviors. When Adelle came out of her bedroom one morning wearing a sweater in the heat of Florida summer, Gary and Nancy protested. She tore it off and threw it in a heap on the floor. "Well, dammit!" she snapped. "I guess I won't wear anything!" She was having an Alzheimer's moment, and they knew to just let it go. Nancy bolts for the phone whenever it rings. Otherwise Adelle will answer and have a reasonable conversation with the caller.

"Who was that?" Nancy typically asks in vain, trying to keep track of things.

"How am I supposed to know?" her mother responds, with a twinge of amused indignation. "I have Alzheimer's disease."

Despite their tenacious hold of the bright side—Adelle can remember how to cook her signature dish, Swedish apple pie with walnuts; she can shower, put on makeup, and dress; she can do simple activities on a computer—they live, nonetheless, with an undercurrent of sadness. Why couldn't she have gotten to the hospital in time to have that third injection before the trial was abruptly halted? What if the researchers had allowed her to sign a release and go on? How much longer can she continue in this relatively high functioning way? Florida is satirically called "God's waiting room" because of the huge population of seniors who have settled there, seeking the steady warmth. Alzheimer's disease is a common problem. A neighbor was symptomatic with it for only five years before requiring constant care. The woman wandered into their house one spring afternoon, unaware of where she was, and had to be led home. Later that day, Stella, who was visiting her parents at the time, opened the door to a back room and found Gary quietly crying.

2

A Friend in the Early Stage: Easy Changes You Can Make

ACKNOWLEDGE THE DIFFICULTY

PEOPLE IN THE EARLY STAGE of Alzheimer's disease can seem okay to friends and relatives. A fifty-eight-year-old man with younger-onset AD complains of feeling pressured by friends who interpret his gaps in memory as carelessness. Although problems may not yet be obvious to others, a diagnosis generally comes after a series of quiet struggles in everyday life with managing finances, remembering commitments and conversations, following directions, keeping track of valued items, and staying on schedule. Some people with early or mild AD report strange, intense bouts of anxiety when they leave home for any length of time. Some have trouble with hand-eye coordination, depth perception, and balance. The first symptoms, while not always consistent, do indicate permanent, debilitating changes in the brain.

Saying to someone with cancer "You look healthy to me; maybe you don't have it" would be insensitive. Don't suggest, similarly, to a friend with AD nothing is wrong. An AD patient must come to terms with the realization that no part of life will remain as before. One of the adjustments friends need to make (not so big in comparison) is to accept the validity of the diagnosis and the resulting inability to control behaviors which may upset and inconvenience others at times. In the initial stages of AD, your friend is both the person you have known and loved and a person confronting the gradual decline of his reasoning power. With this in mind, **refrain** from saying:

- *"I forget things. Everyone does. It's all right."* This remark may seem supportive, but it minimizes the frustration of serious memory loss, which impacts almost every activity of the day.

- *"You need to get out more and try harder. Fight the disease."* Loss of initiative, like memory loss, is one of the warning signs. Many people with AD try to maintain skills and stay active and are unable, despite great effort, to change the course of the disease.[14]

- *"Be positive. Keep doing what you've been doing."* Intervals of depression and discouragement are unavoidable *because* it's not possible to carry on as before.

- *"What you said was [witty, clever, sharp, or insightful]. You're back to your old self!"* A person in the early stage may have the sense of shifting on a day-to-day basis between his reliable brain of the past and the unpredictable brain of the present. There is no going back with permanence to the old self. To suggest otherwise is to make your friend feel he cannot live up to expectations, and reacting with surprise to evidence of continued intelligence is an unintentional putdown. Even though he may have trouble planning ahead, remembering what has just happened and thinking as clearly as before, he is the same person as always in the most important respects and will be for some time—possibly a number of years. This is especially true as physicians become increasingly able to diagnose the disease earlier, before discernible symptoms have appeared.

Kris Bakowski, diagnosed with younger-onset AD, writes an

almost reassuring blog in which she interweaves the typical happenings of her life, refreshingly similar to those of other women her age, with an honest account of her challenges. Here's the unremarkable beginning of one of her posts: "My birthday was this week, and my husband came up with ways to remind me of my advancing age." Kris continues, though, "Seven years ago, when I was diagnosed with Alzheimer's, I didn't think I'd make it to fifty-three, hearing about all of the gloom and doom coming our way. And while that gloom and doom is still out there, I can't let it get to me.[15]

● *"But you're so smart. How could you have Alzheimer's?"* Since the onset of AD is gradual, much more of the brain is intact early on than is not. Instead of downplaying, giving advice, or questioning whether your friend actually has a disease—if he has been competently diagnosed, he almost certainly does—empathize with the feelings that would arise naturally from coping on a daily basis with it:

"This must be frustrating. How can I help?"

"I'm not going anywhere. I'll be here for you."

HELP WITH WORD FINDING

Charles, an engineer with a doctoral degree, sits beside a dining room table cluttered with stacks of unread books and papers. He speaks slowly. "I know my language is into trouble. There's a completely destroyed sense of words being together." Subtle problems with spoken language begin early in AD and become more noticeable with time. Words can no longer be brought to mind with ease and assembled into logical sentences at the spur of the moment. People describe a sensation that the words are there, but mired in a kind of "molasses of the mind." Conversations become halting as familiar words fail to surface at will or are replaced, maddeningly and uncontrollably, with nonsensical substitutions, like *fit* or *fun* for the word *fine*.[16]

It can be tricky to intervene. If you understand, filling in the missing words is not necessary. No one likes to be cut off or have sentences finished by an impatient listener. "Come on, get it out" hand gestures, amusing, maybe, to a person in full control of his speech, are unkind when hesitations are brought about by a neurological condition. When your friend is fumbling and has expressed a desire for help, make suggestions. People with early AD tend to substitute descriptions and homonyms for words they can't recall, which makes the guesswork easier.

When to Supply a Missing Word

Friend: I can't find my...the things you use in cold weather. What are they?

You: A jacket and scarf?

Friend: No, glasses. I mean sleeves. The things for your hands.

You: Gloves? Did you wear gloves today?

Friend: Yes! Gloves. I can't find my gloves.

When to Respond to the Message

Friend: I was going home and couldn't think of how to get there. It was too dark to see the roads. I pulled over and tried to ask some, some of those people who aren't old where my neighborhood is. People who aren't old—darn, what's the word for it? They didn't understand me. I don't know how I figured out which turns to make.

You: That could have been dangerous. Should you have Amelia with you when you're out after dark? Everything looks different during the day. [*Instead of: Let's see, you were driving alone at night, and you got lost. Then you pulled over for directions, and a group of teenagers weren't very helpful because they didn't know what you were talking about. Is that how it happened?*]

Friend: Dear old Amelia, always the worrier. She thinks I shouldn't be driving at all. She won't ride with me now. She sits at home. I get angry at her sometimes. Amelia's a sweetheart, though. I couldn't manage without her.

You: Have you talked with your doctor about driving?

TELL, DON'T ASK, ABOUT THE RECENT PAST

How was your day? What did you think of the program? Can you believe she said that about Sidney last night!? Did you make it out to the polls on Tuesday? What have you been up to lately? We use questions about our daily lives as keys to open the door to conversation without thinking twice. A working hippocampus enables the storage of memories that form the answers to such questions, sifting out volumes of unimportant detail like a coarse screen. Scientists first learned the role of the hippocampus in an experimental operation with a disastrous outcome. In 1953, Yale-trained neurosurgeon William Beecher Scoville used a metal straw to remove much of the hippocampus and medial temporal lobes from the brain of a young man suffering from epilepsy. The man, Henry Molaison, known in medical annals by the initials HM, while largely relieved of seizures, lost the ability to remember anything from one minute to the next. He could only retrieve memories stored before the surgery. Scoville, horrified by the result, ensured through wide publicity that such an operation would never be repeated. He had done to Molaison in minutes what Alzheimer's disease does over the course of years.

> *We use questions as keys to open the door to conversation without thinking twice about it.*

In early AD, the hippocampus is breaking down gradually. Although not a consequence of normal aging, it occurs in some ways like the subtle relinquishments which are a part of ordinary experience: A man doesn't brush a thick head of hair one day and have a sunburned bald spot the next; we move up the ranks of reading glasses slowly; fine wrinkles at forty become a deep crisscrossing map by the mid-sixties. The hippocampus is depredated by AD, but unlike changes so disconcertingly revealed in every pass by a mirror, we cannot accurately gauge how fast this is happening, and the process is more complicated than the loss of hair or skin tone.

To be safe, replace questions about the recent past with statements to which your friend can respond without trying to remember.

Instead of: "How was your weekend?"
Try: "Saturday I went to the farmers market and bought tomatoes."

Instead of: "What did you do at the beach last week?"
Try: "While you were away, Evan drove the car for the first time. Melanie said she was scared to death."

Instead of: "Did you go to the fitness center on Thursday?"
Try: "I see you have a new pair of walking shoes."

GIVE YOUR NAME

Running into a person outside the social setting in which you are accustomed to seeing him can trigger momentary alarm when his name flies out of your mind like an escaped canary. For a person with mild AD, these potentially embarrassing moments may happen more often than not and in the usual places, as well. The difference between the occasional slipups we all experience and dealing with AD is a matter of frequency. Think of tripping on a patch of uneven pavement and being in constant peril of taking a spill because of an arthritic knee. Remind your friend of who you are if he fails to address you by name or seems unsure of his connection to you.

Friend: Hello, how are you?

You: Jack Gibson, Charlie. We were on staff at the hospital together. I'm fine, how are you?

Friend: Of course, I knew that. Good to see you again, Jack.

KEEP EYE CONTACT

Intermittent, lingering eye contact is an almost foolproof way to make a friend feel included, but people abandon this courtesy when caught up in awkwardness, uncertainty or, less diplomatically, in petty egotism. Years back, I had to spend evenings, thankfully not often, with a tedious older physician whose eyes darted around in disinterest when we spoke with each other. Charming to my husband, he treated me like a child or a decorative potted tree, one which annoyingly obscured his view of the rest of the room. People with early AD feel they've become invisible if this kind of encounter becomes common, and frequently it does.

> *Make a point of looking a friend with AD in the eye and speaking directly to him.*

Eye contact is particularly important in groups. Because conversation between several people requires timing and quick thinking, we can unintentionally exclude someone who has trouble with these skills. Now and then, it may not matter. Repeated many times, being left out results in the sense that people no longer value what you have to say, and you've been nudged to the sidelines.

Make a point of looking a friend with AD in the eye and speaking directly to him, the way you would anyone else, especially when you are with others. Avoid, however, the knitted brow and prolonged blank stare in the event of a conversational misfire or lost train of thought. Glance up or sideways, and help your friend get back on track: "Hmm…. We were talking about annoying neighbors, and you were telling me about Mrs. Huckstep's yappy little poodle."

QUESTION TO CLARIFY

When asking personal questions, there are essentially two mistakes: plowing thoughtlessly into another's affairs out of self-indulgent curiosity and being so guarded that valuable opportunities to relieve discomfort or enhance understanding in a relationship are missed. Nosy questions ignore commonly accepted boundaries of privacy and feel like an unjustified intrusion. Barring such topics, when unease begins to stir inside, risk the questions that can help you move beyond it. Otherwise the relationship cannot evolve appropriately with changing circumstances. The uninformed assumptions we make about a person, even a good friend, may lead us into attitudes and behaviors which are confusing and hurtful. An example is the frequently held but false belief that people with early AD are not just as upset by unresolved misunderstandings and social rejections as anyone else.

Kris Bakowski, the blogger with younger-onset AD, writes about her feelings of isolation:

> *It's been said many times that Alzheimer's is a disease of loneliness. Loneliness in the sense that others don't realize what you are going through, loneliness in the sense that people around you don't know how to act or react, so they don't, and loneliness in the fact that you feel all alone.... If you were ever the last one picked in gym class you can probably understand this.*

The strategies that work well everywhere will work also with a friend who has mild dementia—be direct, be open-minded, and ask with sensitivity about what you don't understand. Resist ever firing at your friend the rhetorical question "Don't you remember?" In the early stage, you can let him know tactfully that he has already said or done something: "Yes, you told me that." Instead of: "You said the same thing ten minutes ago. Don't you remember?"

You: Were you able to get the books off the top shelf?

Friend: No, and I was on my hind legs.

You: Hind legs? Do you mean you were on a stepladder?

Friend: I can't believe I said that. I'm always saying things I don't mean. I'm not sure who I am anymore. Crazy words come out of my mouth.

You: You're my good friend. Do you want me to help you out, or does it bug you?

Meeting someone like Kris could go this way:

You: What do you do?

Friend: I'm retired.

You: You look young to be retired.

Friend: I have Alzheimer's disease, younger-onset.

You: [*Without a strange look or an awkward pause*] How long have you had it?

Friend: I was diagnosed several years ago.

You: Alzheimer's is in the news a lot lately. You're not alone.

Friend: I never expected it to happen to me, though.

You: I can understand why. Does it make meeting new people hard?

Friend: I don't remember faces and names. When we see each other again, remind me of who you are.

You: [*Don't hesitate to move on.*] I'm thinking of retiring soon. What do you do since you retired? [*This is different from asking a question which relies exclusively on short-term memory, like "What did you do on Friday?"*

If your friend has trouble answering, and you've given him time to think, drop the question and make a statement: "I'm going to take up golfing."]

RECONSIDER YOUR APPROACH

At times we tend, when frustrated by a problem, to apply repeatedly our original solution to it, but with escalating force. Picture the proverbial American tourist yelling his butchered version of a foreign language to a perplexed local. A "more of the same" tactic works in some cases. Hearing loss is one. Raise your voice, and the person straining to understand is grateful. Shouting at someone who can hear but not quickly process words, often an issue with AD, is like trying to drive a bent nail into oak by hammering harder. Calmly reassess when things begin to go wrong. Be willing to slow down and try something different. Keep in mind that you can make compromises, while your friend may no longer be capable of shifting gears to meet your needs.

You: We have to go. Are you looking for your house keys? Do you want a jacket? Have you fed the cat?

Friend: Don't say anything else! It's aggravating when I can't think and I'm being asked questions. Can you sit down and wait a few more minutes? I can't rush. It only makes things worse.

You: Sure. It won't matter if we're late. I don't know why I'm so stressed about being on time.

Friend: I'm in a fog today, and I was yesterday, too. I tried to make cupcakes for Charlotte's birthday party and left out the sugar. I wish I could have done one small thing for my grandchild.

You: That had to be discouraging. Baking makes a mess. It's bad enough when it turns out well.

Friend: Even the dog was disappointed.

SAY IT STRAIGHTFORWARDLY

When talking with a friend in early AD, try to avoid confusing analogies and metaphors, telling stories that meander in unessential detail and abrupt changes in subject, which can be irritating as conversational habits under the best of circumstances. Stick to one topic at a time and speak concisely.

Instead of: "My granddaughter Frances has had her leg tattooed, and it looks like part of the Rorschach inkblot test. Tattoos like hers, she says, were carved long ago into the faces of South Pacific natives using stone chisels. They must have made a lot of trouble for themselves, smearing ground burnt caterpillars into open wounds and draping their cheeks with wet leaves. I'm surprised the human race has survived its own idiocy. Frances seems hell-bent on driving every adult around her, certainly me and I'm in poor health, completely mad. I cannot believe how permissive my daughter is with her. I didn't let Catherine Jane pierce her ears at that age. And speaking of catastrophes, did you hear about Regina's daughter and the boating accident? Poor Cherie was thrown right off the bow."

Try: "My granddaughter got a tattoo. I'm afraid she is disfigured. I hope the tattoo can be removed if she ever reclaims her sanity."

FOLLOW YOUR FRIEND'S LEAD

At a picnic last summer, several friends and I had spread blankets on a hillside by a lake and were chatting and drinking wine as evening fell. Someone asked, wiping her cheek, "Was that a raindrop?" We looked up, unconcerned. A little later a steady light mist began, but we kept eating brownies and watermelon. Thunder rumbled. As we finally started to cram Tupperware back into the coolers, shake out the blankets and pull on sweatshirts, rain was spattering insistently.

Early Alzheimer's disease is like that storm slipping over the landscape—at first barely noticeable. In the middle and late stages the illness becomes a relentless gale. Unlike the driving wind and heavy rain of a temporary storm, it never lets up. Between the first raindrop and the deluge, there is an interlude that can last for years, when social needs haven't substantially changed. A person who can no longer perform surgery or play bridge may enjoy a relaxed gathering, even if he's unable to take part with ease in conversations involving several people.

> *Early Alzheimer's disease is like that storm slipping over the landscape—at first barely noticeable.*

However, AD becomes progressively more conspicuous, mainly due to problems with language: repeating oneself, using descriptive phrases for common words, forgetting what has been recently heard, and odd verbal mistakes. Silence can thus be a coping strategy. While including your friend through eye contact, honor his choice of not speaking over the possibility of self-consciousness, if that option seems safest. Let him determine how much he participates.

ADJUST FOR DAILY SHIFTS

The day-to-day degree of difficulty in AD is unpredictable, depending to an extent on physical and environmental factors such as rest, nutrition, and even, according to some, fluctuations in barometric pressure. If the disease started out with an unmistakable onslaught of symptoms we might be more afraid of it, but we would be less inclined to rationalize it away. Rather, it begins stealthily, like decay in a hidden corner of the eaves of a house. On the better days, a person in early AD will be more able to think and make connections. He is experiencing memory *lapses* at first, encouraging—when memory does snap into place—the temptation to deny that anything unusual is happening. Robert, the therapist with younger-onset AD, said he intermittently had no idea where he was or what was going on as the disease crept into his own awareness, but his confusion lasted just a few minutes. "I'm all right," he told himself. "Everyone loses the way sometimes, and I remember where I'm headed now." Robert admitted his memory loss only when it became apparent to his wife and children.

With a friend in the early stage, adjust for the frequent changes of Alzheimer's. On a good day, your friend may seem to have nothing wrong. On a bad day, he may be frustrated, repetitive, irritable, and unable to focus on your needs and feelings. He's having too much trouble wrestling with his own. During these periods try not to hold against him what he says or neglects to say. Think of it as you would an unexpected rainstorm. He can neither help nor remember the bad days, and you can imagine the difficulty of having thoughts and intentions slip from your mind before you can act on them. Your friend is no more in control of the disease than you are of the weather.

TAKE CARE OF TRUST

Relationships are contingent on the stability of behaviors and attitudes demonstrated over time. As one person in a relationship loses the ability to initiate and respond as usual, established patterns re-evolve, either consciously or by default. The old rules no longer apply, since those heartfelt talks in which expectations are made explicit may not be remembered by both of the people involved. This change doesn't revoke the importance of basic trust. When his confidence has been shaken to the core, your friend needs, more than ever, the reassurance of his loved ones' continued belief in him as a competent person, capable of contributing and talking openly about his condition.

Along with the frustration of being unable to fully control words, which can escape the lips like horses through an open gate, a person in the early stage may be painfully aware that cherished relationships have begun to take on an altogether different, less intimate dynamic. A man in early AD, visiting friends a thousand miles from his home, told me in clear terms how much he wanted to ask his wife, "Why haven't we had sex since my diagnosis?" He wanted to ask his son, "Why haven't you called me 'Dad' since my diagnosis?" But he wasn't able to speak frankly with the people he loved. He feared that if he tried, the words would not come out as intended, and he couldn't face the prospect of the jumbled, hurtful exchange that might take place. Instead of addressing delicate issues, he brooded in silent resentment as his wife and son talked in hushed tones about him, presuming he wouldn't hear, understand, or care.

It requires patience and flexibility to nurture trust in a relationship when one member of the pair must adapt to involuntary changes in the other. Think of this analogy: If you had to build a house at a place prone to earthquakes, you would make the design basic and close to the ground, not a big complicated structure on stilts. Speak explicitly and without elaboration, realizing relationship discussions can't move nimbly around the emotional map, the way they may have in the past. Here are two examples; the first doesn't work, the second does:

A Muddled Message

Friend: It bothers me when you talk about me when I'm standing nearby, like I can't hear you. I'm not deaf.

You: This is hard for me, too. I'm irritated when you forget we've made plans. I don't see why you can remember some things and not what we've decided to do together.

Friend: I can't make myself remember what I want to. Why don't you call and remind me before you leave your house?

A Clear Message

Friend: It bothers me when you talk about me when I'm standing nearby, like I can't hear you. I'm not deaf.

You: I'm sorry. I didn't know I was doing that.

Friend: People are treating me like I don't have opinions or anything worthwhile to say. I do, and I can talk for myself.

You: I'll be sure to talk directly to you from now on. But as long as we're bringing up complaints, I have one, too.

Friend: With what?

You: When you forget our plans, it throws off my schedule. Can you write yourself a note, or should I call before I come over?

Friend: It's better to call. I'm having trouble writing now.

LEND A SUBTLE HAND

Have you ever had to ask for help paying a bill while people stood in line behind you at the cash register? Forgotten whether or not you've ordered at a restaurant? Had trouble finding your way back to the table? Drawing a mental blank in the midst of everyday activities is one of the first signs of AD. As mentioned, these setbacks fluctuate in the beginning. Some days, a person in the early stage can manage independently, and overattentiveness from a companion may be irritating. It would be to most of us. People resent being smothered, mothered, or treated as if inept. Rather than assuming your friend will always want help, decide together on a way he can easily tell you his needs from one time to the next. This may be accomplished by redefining the standard answer to "How are you today?"

"Fine," meaning: "I'm having a pretty good day. If I need your help, I'll ask for it."

"Not the best," meaning: "I'm frustrated. Help me out and don't take what I say or do personally. This is one of the bad days."

To get an idea of the support that may be necessary in case of "not the best," try an experiment. Imagine being given these directions to the restroom in a public place: "Go up the parth and moof to the rigfap on bruck. It's the third door on the flirtch."

"I'm sorry," you stammer. "What did you say?"

The very busy host looks annoyed and repeats, "To the parth, by the rigfap on the flirtch."

You would feel entitled to your own annoyance and call into question, perhaps, the host's sobriety. Nonsense words with insufficient context are impossible to decipher. But what if you realized you were trying to make sense of the language, rapidly or impatiently spoken, that you've used your whole life? Anticipate greater frustration on "not the best" days and unobtrusively offer help:

- *"I'm having the Greek salad, or here's pasta with chicken. Do either of those sound good to you?"*

- *"I'll figure out the bill. Why don't we split it evenly?"*

- *"I'm going downstairs to wash my hands. Would you like to come, too?"*

- *"This shopping center is crowded. Do you want to go to a quieter place?"*

FACE THE DRIVING DILEMMA

Many people in the early stage of Alzheimer's disease continue to drive; driving skills may remain intact for a considerable time after the diagnosis. The privilege of driving and the independence it represents are difficult to relinquish, and disagreements between family members over when it should stop for safety's sake sometimes cause hard feelings. As a friend or relative, however, you can at any point, whether others have made the same decision or not, take on the role of designated driver, particularly if you've noticed changes in your friend's driving—slower than normal reaction time and driving speed, inappropriate stopping or lane changes, problems with directions, failing to notice traffic lights and signs. At an opportune moment, you should mention these observations to the caregiver. Avoid, however, being drawn into an emotional, spur-of-the-moment confrontation with your friend. Try a polite broken-record approach, a gentle way of diverting conflict and of removing the pressure to explain yourself at risk of a friend's hurt or anger. Here is an example:

You: I'll pick you up at seven o'clock.

Friend: No, I'll drive.

You: Thanks, but I'll pick you up. I don't mind. [*Instead of: I don't want to drive with you anymore. I'm sorry, but it makes me nervous.*]

Friend: I can still drive, you know. I have a valid license. In fifty years, I've never had an accident. Why does it bother you?

You: I realize you still drive, but I want to. Can I pick you up at seven? [*Instead of: It bothers me because you have dementia.*]

Friend: I'm the same person I was six months ago. I drive as well as anybody else.

You: [*Responding to the underlying issue*] Of course you're the same person, and I care about you the same way. You're my favorite aunt! But I always like to be the driver. I'm really looking forward to trying the new restaurant with you. Is seven o'clock convenient?

MAKE COMFORTING MOVES

Rabbi David Wolpe, in his wise book, *Making Loss Matter*, tells the story of a man who lived in a village in Eastern Europe. Scathed by two World Wars, the people of the village were, for the most part, hardened and cold toward outsiders. One man, though, was outgoing, accepting, welcoming. A visiting rabbi, rebuffed by everyone else, asked of this man, "Why? What makes you different?"

> *The man smiled. "I know why, and I can tell you when it happened. I am an old man, and I have lived in this town my entire life. And I recall one night before the First World War, a rumor swept through the town that there would be a pogrom. We were told that the Cossacks were coming, and they would loot and pillage and destroy. So all the parents from the whole town gathered up all the children and brought us to the rabbi's house....*
>
> *"I was curled up in a small corner of the rabbi's study. He thought I was sleeping, but it was bitter cold—I could not sleep. He came up behind me and slipped his cloak off his shoulders, and he laid it over me and said, 'Good child, sweet child.'*
>
> *"You know," said the man to Rabbi Carlebach, "it has been seventy-five years since the rabbi spread his coat over me—but it still keeps me warm."*
>
> *In the midst of loss, in the cold night, with the threat of destruction hanging over everyone's head, the rabbi made a gesture of love. For the rest of that child's life, he was different because he knew that fear and pain and even loss were not all. Because he knew that we cannot escape losing but we can keep each other warm.[17]*

Sometimes there are no words. The best response is to take a friend in your arms and give the kind of comfort and closeness that transcends words. Imagine a friend saying, "I've been diagnosed with Alzheimer's disease. My wife and I have been crying for days. There aren't any tears left. We are terrified."

Think of the difference between hugging your friend or putting your hand on his arm, saying only "How can I help?" and blurting out a misguided condolence, which would do nothing more than add to the distress:

- *"Being forgetful isn't so bad. Everyone forgets things."*

- *"That can't be right. Have you gotten a second medical opinion? I thought I had Alzheimer's, and it turned out to be menopause."*

- *"Have faith. Be strong. We're not given more than we can bear."*

- *"You're healthy in other ways; that's a plus."*

- *"I'm sure they'll find a cure. Try not to worry."*

- *"I don't see anything wrong with you."*

SHAPE A NEW RELATIONSHIP

In *The Seven Habits of Highly Effective People*, Stephen Covey says to consider the give and take of friendships in terms of bookkeeping in an emotional account. We make investments by doing things that increase a friend's trust; we make withdrawals in acts of thoughtlessness and betrayal. A strong positive balance keeps the relationship viable. This system is based on equivalence in the "currency" each person offers—the ability to initiate and plan enjoyable events, reciprocate, act on important discussions, make amends and forgive, each of which is contingent on memory.

In your relationship with a friend in early AD, imagine instead sailing on the open sea without a ledger of rights and wrongs. Sailors can't plan far ahead; they must work with the wind and waves of the moment. They can't march off the boat in a huff over a brewing storm. They enjoy the sun when it is shining and the sea when it is calm, understanding the inevitability of rapid change. With a loved one in the early stage of dementia, you are more a sailor than a banker. Forgotten plans, one-sided conversations, and turns of sudden anger or frustration are part of a journey, always worthwhile in its larger contexts of humanity and compassion, if challenging from the standpoints of ease and traditional reciprocity. In working out the changes in the relationship:

Remain in contact. You can help by continuing to include your friend in activities he would normally enjoy and in which he can safely participate.

Be flexible. You may have to cancel plans at the last minute. He cannot override his state of mind. You'd make the same concession for someone with an upset stomach or a migraine headache. Think in advance of an alternative for the time you've set aside: "It's okay if you don't feel like going, John. I can either stay for a visit, or I have errands I can run." The concepts of date, day of the week, and hour of the day become hazy. Always call a short while ahead with a reminder of plans you've made and tell the caregiver, too. Build in extra time. As indicated in an earlier dialogue (*Reconsider Your Approach*, page 38), hurrying is never a good idea.

Support strengths. Faith, humor, optimism, perseverance, and courage are among the character traits of many people with mild AD and caregivers alike. Acknowledge and encourage these strengths, without reproaching your friend when they aren't clearly in evidence on a given day. "Cheer up!" "Don't let it get the best of you," "Be brave," and other such exhortations tend to raise hackles when coming from a person who doesn't face the same set of trying circumstances. Along with the unwelcome changes, there can still be joy, and the depth of love and commitment often present in caregiving and other relationships is heartwarming. When your friend seems down, try saying your own version of the Bill Withers classic, "Lean on Me."

- *"I'll be here for you; you'd do the same for me."*

- *"You're my friend. I'm here to stay."*

- *"Thinking of the future is hard, but I'm with you now, and I will be then."*

"I'm a Care Partner Now?"
Help at the Beginning

ACKNOWLEDGE THE REALITIES

"I'M A CARE PARTNER? What? My [*husband, wife, father, sister...*] doesn't really need a care partner or caregiver,* not yet, anyway." A person does not suddenly snap into the role of caregiver, barring an incapacitating stroke or injury, any more than a patient suddenly has Alzheimer's: It happens gradually, over years. But the label, "dementia caregiver," and an understanding of what caregiving will ultimately mean—caring, literally, for every aspect of a loved one's existence— become shockingly real after the diagnosis of AD has been confirmed. Alice, a new care partner, well-dressed and poised beside her successful husband, is unsettled by her anticipation of changes that will occur in him and within their relationship as the disease evolves. "I don't know, from one day to the next," she says, "what [ability] he'll lose that will never come back. We have to look ahead and plan. We know what is coming, for the most part, and it's not easy to face."

---

* Caregivers are sometimes referred to as care partners, especially in the beginning, when the assistance required by the patient is limited. The terms are synonymous.

People unfamiliar with this situation, who may see only superficial evidences of lifestyle, can miss how challenging it is to manage these steadily accumulating losses. I was with a caregiver in her living room, when she reached across the coffee table for an embroidered knick-knack. "So What?" was stitched against a cream background bordered in a frilly blue ruffle. She uses the question as a reminder to let go of things that don't really matter in light of her husband's dementia, and one of these is the pang she feels when friends comment, "I can't see anything wrong with him at all." She replies, "Well, there is—quite a lot." She understands her friends don't mean to be hurtful with the observation, and that from their perspective, it's accurate. Her husband, well into mid-stage Alzheimer's at the time of our interview, could no longer drive a car, remember his children's names or make a sandwich, but he retained many of the social graces of his former life as a corporate executive.

Some people with AD can be as charming as ever in a short conversation, even after communication with immediate family members has downgraded to confused, repetitive exchanges. No matter how reassuring it is to think differently, Alzheimer's disease is a terminal condition that leads to complete impairment. This fact cannot be called into question with legitimate hope of a breakthrough cure soon or the possibility of an inaccurate medical evaluation.

When a friend tells you of a spouse, parent, or close loved one's diagnosis:

* *Resist the temptation to report your contradictory perceptions.* "She can't have Alzheimer's! Last week she told me the whole recipe for beef stew. It has fourteen ingredients. Are you sure? I think they're wrong."

* *Don't rush into an overly optimistic conjecture.* "Scientists are finding treatments for everything now. In a few years, new medications should be available, and your husband will be fine."

- *Gloom and speechlessness are not comforting.* "Oh, no. She doesn't, does she? Alzheimer's disease is worse than death."

- *Levity is inappropriate.* "Well, there you go. Payback for the grief you gave your mother when you were a kid!"

- *Refrain from speculating about the cause of the disease in hopes of freeing yourself from personal worry.* "Did one of your grandparents have Alzheimer's? Your father drank too much, didn't he? I wonder if his weight had anything to do with it. Do you think you might get it, too?"

- *Don't brush off the diagnosis.* "Well, how old is she, anyway? Isn't she almost eighty? That's pretty old. We'll probably be losing our own minds by then."

This is a safe way to respond:

- *Briefly, sincerely express sympathy.* "That news had to be very hard to hear."

- *If you have friends in common, inquire whether other people are being told. Some feel strongly that medical information should be kept private.* "Do you and Philip want anyone else to know at this point? Should I tell the [book group, parish, tai chi class, quilting club], so they'll be sensitive to what you and your family are going through?"

- *Ask about your friend's welfare, but avoid drawing your own conclusions.* "How are you holding up?" Instead of: "You look [tired, worried, pale, depressed, or still so amazingly cheerful]."

- *Offer your companionship.* "We're having a quiet supper on Sunday evening. Would the two of you like to join us?"

As the months and years go by, and problems become more entrenched, both the caregiver and the person with dementia will be conscious of every loss and altered ability. To outsiders, the disease may remain largely hidden. Should the caregiver mention a difficulty that doesn't seem so significant from your perspective, think about the broader implications and don't make light of it. A person with AD who can no longer assemble a seven-layer cake from scratch will in time be unable to button her own blouse. No one suffers for lack of a fancy dessert (no need to point that out), but the future implied by such relatively minor losses is a tremendously troubling prospect.

BE AN ANCHOR

Relationships are tested by time. Ideally, adult children and aging parents become enduring friends with a long and unique background. Friendships bound by specific settings, like work or school, tend to peter out when there are no longer mutual problems to solve and prearranged hours to share. We expect our carefully chosen adult relationships to evolve with the major developments in our lives, yet serve as predictable touchstones to which we can return for a sense of stability.

With a diagnosis of AD or any progressive dementia, the fear is not so much of the unknown but the known: A spouse, parent, or partner who's loved more, perhaps, than anyone else in the world will be transformed by AD. The shared history and dreams will be lost; the quirky, quick-witted, strong, irascible, creative personality will be lost and the bond as intimate companion supplanted by that of caregiver. As with Willa and Bert, whose story is told in chapter 10, the downturn need not portend a loss of love itself, but the expression of that love will be different.

In the 1990s, Julian Davidson, a professor at Stanford, was diagnosed with younger-onset AD. Within a relatively short period, he was unable to comprehend his own research articles. His wife, Ann, wrote a touching memoir about their experience. She describes how hard it was to witness her husband's transformation from a highly respected scientist to a mentally disabled adult in need of her undivided attention, saying she felt "abandoned, inch by inch, in slow motion."[18] I heard a similar story one morning in the living room of a former financial officer, a distinguished man sitting in a wing chair with his dog at his side. His wife and caregiver told me they had met half a century earlier at a tea dance when he was thirteen and she was twelve. That evening, he precociously informed her, "You know, I may marry you one day!" And he did. They lived a full, rewarding life with children, travel, and equally successful careers until about seven years ago, when she noticed that her husband was forgetting appointments and important events. She received a major business award, and he never showed up for the banquet. "We had talked about it less than an hour before." She looked back on the incident, seemingly unable, still, to believe it. "I didn't know what to think." A lifelong athlete, he couldn't keep his balance. One afternoon he stumbled and fell down the stairs in their home.

They were approaching their fortieth anniversary, and given their mutual love of entertaining, she naturally thought of having a party to celebrate, despite his growing problems with memory loss. "We'd talk about it, and he wouldn't say anything. Then we'd talk about it again, and he wouldn't say anything," she remembers, all too well. "We wound up going alone to our beach house. On the way there I mentioned the anniversary, and he asked, 'What anniversary?' I broke down in tears."

ROLES CHANGE RADICALLY with Alzheimer's disease. "We've been married fifty-two years," said Betsy, a homemaker whose husband was diagnosed with early stage AD. "I've been reading so many books about these wonderful, brilliant people it happens to, and I'm almost convinced these are the only ones who are written about. My husband played at Wimbledon. He has a doctorate. He's that typical story of an unbelievably bright, energetic person. He just...." Her voice trailed off for a moment, then she looked up with resolve. "On the other hand, he took care of me for fifty years. Now I'm going to take care of him."

Particularly during the adjustment to this new and troubling circumstance, the caregiver needs other important people in her life to be calm and dependable. Consider this analogy: If you've ever watched racehorses going to the gate, there are always a few plunging wildly around with a jockey in a colorful cap and jersey bobbing in the saddle like a cork on a wave. Alongside there's a plodding pony who gives the impression that the world could split open, and he would hop quietly over the crack. The emotional upheaval of the disease is like the racehorse; the clinging jockey is the caregiver; and you, the close friend or relative, must at times be the pony. A woman dealing simultaneously with the grief of her mother's protracted battle with AD and a daughter caught in the hormonal tempest of adolescence said she was aware of being short tempered but too stressed to keep herself in check. At one point, her daughter shouted back at her, "You're a maniac!"

"And I was," she confesses. "I was." Able in that instant to see the impact on her own family of her unresolved feelings about her mother, she began to rely on friends and a therapist to help her stay more grounded. When a person's world is crashing, she counts on her friends to hold steady and keep in normal contact while she makes the necessary psychological and emotional compensations. Here are a few suggestions for how to do this:

Be sensitive in conversation. As a caregiver worries about how she'll cope with the changes in her loved one and lifestyle, her optimism and ability to rejoice in another's good fortune may be at a low ebb. Listening to the details of happy vacation plans or a terrific retirement can cause a private dive into a sense of loss. Be conscious of your friend's challenges. You can step freely in and out of the dementia patient's world. Your friend cannot. She needs your compassion and sometimes your restraint. Caregiving is not without rewards, and as one caregiver told me, it's a steady opportunity for personal growth. Not many of us, however, would choose the experience.[19]

Be flexible. The unpredictability of AD makes time management difficult for a stay-at-home caregiver. Leaving the house is not a simple turnkey operation, and unanticipated holdups are par for the course. Allow a cushion of time in your planning, or call ahead. The caregiver may need to cancel at the last minute. As mentioned at the end of chapter 2, have other ideas in mind for your time.

Continue to invite your friend out. Don't be dissuaded by frequent regrets. Assume, unless you're told to the contrary, she appreciates being considered and will join you when possible. Make clear whether the person with AD is included: "We're having a few people over for a casual dinner on the porch. Can you and Terry come, or just you, if he'd rather not? Either way is fine, but we would miss seeing Terry." Or: "Can you join us for a ladies night out? Will Terry be okay staying alone for an evening?"

Forego the expectation of being invited back. Caregivers may occasionally entertain or plan a get together, but more often, dealing with the inevitable shifts (*How will Terry feel tomorrow? Will it be one of the easier days, or will something go wrong?*) precludes thinking ahead with confidence. The finer order of grace must prevail. Keep your friend in your life because of the relationship you've built together, not because she's in a position to match your hospitality. Caregiving to a loved one with dementia ultimately becomes a consuming responsibility that seldom gives openings for social connection. A committed friend can have a considerable impact on this part of the problem.

CARE FOR THE CAREGIVER

A caregiver preoccupied by a parent or spouse's dementia can't always be the fun and witty person she may have been before this disease came to the foreground. In the turmoil of real adversity, no matter what the reason, the challenge is to keep from being frankly depressing. Staying upbeat is like trying to swim wearing a pair of mud boots.

I found this to be true in my own experience. Shortly after losing my husband, I went to Colorado to stay for a while with my closest friend, who had turned her basement bedroom into a comforting haven for me, choosing new cushions and a bedcover with warm tones. Suzanne and I had grappled together with the minor torments and triumphs of graduate school and a decade of life changes, including her move to this place, 1500 miles from where we had lived for several years just a few blocks apart. Unacquainted with the dramatic weather that rolls over the Rockies in early spring, I hadn't planned to rent a car. I rode around the county in cold sweeping winds on a purple bicycle I had dismantled and shipped from home.

One morning snow was falling so heavily, I accompanied Suzanne to run errands instead of pedaling down the six-mile-long trail that connected her neighborhood to the main part of town. Between stops we went for coffee, and as we sat wedged in a crowded cafe, the snow began to melt and course in rivulets through beds of blooming tulips outside the window. I was determined to be passably cheerful. I smiled and chatted in pace with the people around us, who seemed happy and animated in the unexpected sunlight. Later in the afternoon, Suzanne pulled into the parking lot of her office to dash inside the building for some papers. As soon as she shut the car door behind her, the emotions I had held back broke through. I sobbed uncontrollably into my winter gloves and wiped my face with the nubby wool. Returning, she settled into her seat and looked at me for a long moment. She reached over, slipped her hand in mine and said, "I will never leave you, Mary." Six words—knitted immediately into my heart. I hear them now as a plain and clear statement of love that hasn't faded in the unfolding of subsequent years. There are few more powerful messages one friend can give another than the promise of presence through the bad times as well as the good. Suzanne is an All-Weather Friend.

PART TWO

Mid-Stage

4

Neal's Story

Once he fell in the middle of the night, and after I had gotten him up, he said, "You're extremely good to me. Extremely good. Who are you?"

I said, "Well, I'm your wife. Do you know my name?"

He said, "Janet?"

(She laughed as she told the story.) Janet's not the one changing his clothes. Whoever Janet was, she's long since gone! You do get the occasional compliment, but in the next moment, he wants to know who I am or where he is. It's the small things that get you down. Life is in seconds. He'll think clearly for seconds, and then it's over.

We agree in support group that the marriages end. The partnership is gone. You stay because you care but not because anything comes back to you with any kind of uplift. All the sorts of things that would be part and parcel of my life are gone.

— CATHRYN

CATHRYN MET NEAL when she was a young woman, living in her native London. He was a widower, almost fifty. He had climbed the ranks of a corporation and was negotiating its post Second World War expansion into Japan, Australia, Europe, India, and Iceland. The marriage took Cathryn to the four corners of the world. She gave birth to their only child, a son, in Switzerland. A family album shows the Neal of decades past in boardrooms and corporate parties. The photographs could be frames cut from a classic 1950s movie. They had an exciting life, made possible by his negotiating prowess and skill as an analyst. Her favorite times were summers they spent salmon fishing in a thatch roofed hut on the banks of a Norwegian river. The water was no more than waist deep, she said, and so clear you could see the fish running like bold patterns of a tribal rug. They lived for weeks on wild strawberries and the salmon they caught.

> *A family album shows the Neal of decades past in boardrooms and corporate parties.*

CURIOUSLY, THE FIRST inkling of Neal's disease was his inexplicable reluctance to travel. To Cathryn's consternation, he called off trips, from the Outer Banks to Montreal, seemingly undeterred by the stiff financial penalties often levied on last-minute cancellations. This man, who had spent the better part of his career effortlessly shifting between conveyances and living quarters on every continent, now abhorred being away from home for more than two days. Eventually he began to thumb rides around the neighborhood; he stopped strangers on the street to tell jokes a six-year-old might find funny, maybe reaching back for the dry clever wit that had disarmed the corporate world. Indulgent neighbors picked him up and brought him home repeatedly. Less than two years after he had rashly cancelled a trip to the Pyrenees, Cathryn found her husband dripping blood in the bathroom from a failed attempt to shave. He could not remember to flush used toilet paper, dropping it to the floor; he would take food from his mouth and put it back into the serving containers; he had flung a dish at her in anger; he couldn't remember the names of children from his first marriage. The following year, he could not tie his own shoes.

The term *moderate*, sometimes used interchangeably with *middle* to designate this stage, must seem ironic to caregivers. The amount of help needed by a person who can no longer bathe, dress, or stay at home alone for an hour or two is not moderate. As the disease spreads through regions of the brain that control language, judgment, reasoning, emotional control and sensory processing, caregiving can seem more like wrestling with an irrational stranger who lacks any understanding of how to meet the most basic needs.

In the mid-stage, Neal recognized Cathryn well enough now and then to threaten her with divorce when he was irate and refer to himself as "your stupid husband" in frustration. After he had wet and soiled the carpets, the floor, the bed and his clothes, she persuaded him to wear incontinence pads, which she then found strewn around the house and stuffed in drawers. He hoarded bits of chicken and vegetables and hid them under the toilet brush in the bathroom. He tagged along with her constantly, clearing his throat and asking questions: *Who is the President? Who is the cleaning lady? Where does our son live? What does he do? Did they drop the atomic bomb on Germany? Are the Pakistanis fighting the Israelis?*

The hippocampus enables the interpretation of time and spatial relationships, and once it goes, even the circumscribed world of retirement becomes a senseless maze. Within a seemingly short period, early stage difficulties driving a known route may transform to the more terrible prospect of losing the way between the bathroom and bedroom in one's own home. Exhibiting typical mid-stage patterns of behavior, Neal was restless through the evening and into nighttime. He seemed equally bewildered morning and evening, reaching his most lucid state, such as it was, around midday. Before he left to spend the rest of his life at a nursing home, he often muddled around the house during the predawn hours while Cathryn was sleeping. She awakened one night to find him downstairs sitting at the dining room table in the dark, dressed, expecting dinner to be served. Bleary-eyed from a sedative, she had to lead him back to his bedroom, change him into his pajamas, and hope he stayed in bed. Before daybreak another morning, he roused her by opening the front door to linger at the threshold, contemplating the silent streets of the neighborhood. "What are you doing?" she asked, again having groped her way to the foyer from a deep sleep.

"Well," he explained, "I'm new in the area, and I need to get to know it."

The middle of the night is not the only odd time caregivers must remain vigilant about the possibility of erratic, potentially dangerous behavior. With silverware and table accessories forming so many parts and pieces of a puzzle, mealtimes can be as confusing to a person with AD as it once was to be lost downtown in rush hour traffic. Familiar objects (pebbles, detergent, the soil of potted plants, toothpaste, holiday decorations) are sometimes mistaken for food. Books on caregiving have many tips: Place one type of food on the plate at a time, set out only a fork or make foods that can be eaten neatly with the fingers, take the salt and pepper shakers off the table. Use plastic tablecloths, lidded cups, and aprons.

> ✒ *Mealtimes can be as confusing to a person with AD as it once was to be lost downtown in rush hour traffic.*

The last meal of the day, which for most of us ritualistically divides work from the relaxation of evening, can become a rigor that underscores a harsh reality of caregiving: Without another person's help, there is never a break. From the mid-stage on, caregiving is a job that takes place seamlessly from day to day, like continual shifts, one tagged on another, in nursing. In many cases, it goes on without thanks. Because Alzheimer's disease disrupts the perception of hunger and thirst, a person in mid-stage may crave food minutes after eating or refuse to eat at standard intervals, undermining even the concept of a dinner hour. Neal, a member during retirement of a society that met for a monthly evening meal and discussion of literature, abruptly lost his table manners. He swigged sherry straight from the bottle, took his false teeth out at the table, and blew his nose in his napkin. He stuffed food into his pockets, angrily threatening to hit his wife if she tried to dispose of it. "The whole performance revolted me," said Cathryn, a professional actress in younger years. "Eventually I thought I couldn't bear any more of it."

ROUTINES OF DAILY LIVING, taken for granted and done mindlessly from the time of childhood, are a series of baffling ordeals. Cathryn borrowed a shower seat and began to wash Neal when it became apparent he no longer knew how to clean himself. Cathryn is a slender woman, about five feet, five inches tall. Neal was then a robust man, strong even at his advanced age. He wasn't always easy to wash.

He was sick with vomiting and diarrhea several years after his diagnosis with AD, and Cathryn had to take him to the hospital. The typical emergency room is a place of trial and tribulation for caregivers, who must placate an uncomprehending adult with the demeanor of a frightened, fretful child throughout a lengthy wait in a bedlam of noise and confusion. Cathryn finally left him there, still vomiting, sometime after midnight. Back home the next morning, Neal, recovered and smelling to high heaven, reacted violently to her suggestion of a shower and change of clothes. "He shook me," she said incredulously. "You know how they shake babies to kill them, back-and-forth and side-to-side? I was really scared!" Fortunately their son was visiting at the time and came to the rescue. He stood over his father, making use of his own intimidating physique, and ordered him upstairs to the bathroom. Neal acquiesced. "All right," he said, realizing the disadvantage in his immediate position. "But I'm cutting you out of my will."

"What can you do, but laugh?" Cathryn asked. "We just fell about! So we got him clean, but those are the extraordinary moments."

As with many caregivers, Cathryn has learned to find a silver lining of humor not totally obscured by the brunt of the storm. While AD causes a nonstop regression in language and self-care abilities, this process is not happening in the absence of very unchildlike social sensibilities, which can remain illogically fixed in long-term memory like endnotes separated from the related content. Such incongruence can make for some amusing moments, no matter how tragic the overall situation, and as Cathryn concluded, what can you do but laugh? A husband taking care of his wife was helping her fasten her bra in front of a large mirror. She looked at her sagging breasts and observed with regret, "Oh, they've gotten so flat."

As with many caregivers, Cathryn has learned to find a silver lining of humor not totally obscured by the brunt of the storm.

Meaning to comfort her, he replied, "They may be flat now, but I remember when we could stand martini glasses on them."

She wheeled and gave him a frosty stare. "I don't know *who* you are," she exclaimed. "But you shouldn't be talking to me like that!"

DURING MID-STAGE, it may become evident, as it did to Cathryn, that home care will not always be feasible. Placement in a nursing home is the most common alternative. To the well-off or well-insured, this decision poses serious considerations related to choosing between options and the common emotional consequence of guilt, often deeply felt at the prospect of relinquishing the care of a loved one to an institution. To those of more limited means, it can threaten a financial disaster. The average annual cost of a skilled nursing home exceeds the median household income, as reported by the Census Bureau, by more than twenty thousand dollars. A caregiver in Connecticut, who built a cottage next to her own home and hired a round-the-clock aide to care for her mother, worked full time to pay for it. There was, she said, not one dime left over, and her mother lived into her nineties.

For many people, the only alternative is a custom modification of the house to prolong the time caregiving can be provided without professional assistance. This, at best, is a daunting task. Consider the burden of creating a safe environment for someone apt to wander out the front door in the middle of a freezing night wearing only pajamas. Someone who cannot remember how to coordinate the motions of walking and may stumble over any small item of furniture, throw rug, or shoe left out of place. Someone perfectly capable of rummaging around in the laundry room and opening a gallon of bleach but incapable of understanding what not do with it. For starters, being on guard can involve installing alarms on doors leading outside, putting child proof locks on cabinets, removing the knobs from the stove, concealing electrical cords, turning the oven off at the circuit box when not in use, labeling doors to the bed and bathrooms, marking frequently traveled routes around the house with large arrows, rendering inaccessible the many sharp or dangerous objects common in any household, and completely eliminating clutter.

Further adaptations may become necessary as natural light diminishes at the end of each day. Do you remember how, as a child, you may have been frightened by the distorted shadows in a darkened room? How the dresser looked large and hulking, and the rumpled clothes on the chair seemed more like a sleeping animal? To a person in the middle years of Alzheimer's disease, dusk can be a time of heightened anxiety due to fatigue, the clinking and clattering around dinnertime, and shadows in the dimming light. Imagine catching sight of yourself in a mirror and thinking an intruder has broken into the house or hearing voices on television and wondering why strangers are in your den. Some caregivers resort to draping blankets over mirrors, the television screen, and other reflective surfaces at night.

Cathryn considered making adjustments to the house to ensure Neal's safety as his mind continued to collapse, but after suffering a minor stroke herself, she situated him in an assisted living facility. The decision to place a loved one outside the home, however wrenching, is often spurred by the caregiver's health needs. The stress of caregiving would tax the reserves of the most stalwart among us, and for Cathryn, the already strenuous physical demands were compounded by her husband's size. She could not lift him or easily move his arms and legs around to dress him. And she would scarcely have been able to defend herself, were he ever to fly into an irrational rage—a hard truth to face about a man addressed by his devoted longtime secretary as "my dear, dear, dear Mr. Wood."

> *The decision to place a loved one outside the home, however wrenching, is often spurred by the caregiver's health needs.*

As mentioned earlier, mid-stage AD is sometimes compared to early childhood, when tantrums, imaginary friends, and separation anxiety are normal. If a little person with rosy cheeks and large eyes sits down and yells "NO!" our annoyance is tempered by the realization such displays of immaturity will diminish over time. When an eighty-year-old, who retains memories of the Depression but has lost both emotional control and the capacity to understand his environment, yells in red-faced paranoia that you have stolen his money, staying calm can be a much greater challenge.

The person with dementia may no longer be able to relate to either his caregiver or you, except as someone to whom he assigns a mistaken identity based on fragments of remaining memory. You may become his wife, a close friend from early adulthood, his son or his daughter. He may be happy to see you because in the moment he is convinced you are a neighbor he liked as a child. To the caregiver, you are a connection to the outside world—to normality and life before Alzheimer's.

A WHILE AGO I ACCOMPANIED CATHRYN TO VISIT NEAL at his nursing home. He sat at a table with five other people. Each had a picture of a bear torn from a coloring book. Crayons were scattered about.[20] *Oh, you beautiful doll,* cheerfully babbled from a CD player. *You great big beautiful doll. Can I put my arms around you? Gee! I'm just so glad I found you....*

"Neal!" Cathryn implored. "Neal, color the bear's other foot. He can't have one white foot! Can he, Neal?"

A woman sitting next to Neal giggled. "Robbie?" she said, obviously addressing him. "It's the one you can't find, Robbie. The one you can't find. This isn't yellow, Robbie, like I wanted it to be." She turned to Cathryn. "I need a hankie."

Cathryn rummaged in her purse. "Here, it's a real one. It won't tear."

The woman hesitated, caught in a momentary dilemma. "No, no, no. I can't take this of yours, or maybe I'll just wash it for you, before I give it back."

"All right, you do that."

I was dismayed to see Elaine, whose story follows in chapter 12, slumped in a chair across the room, the side of her face flat against the table in front of her. Her hair had grown several inches and hung in unruly waves about her shoulders. An aide gave her arm a shake. "Are you sleepy?" she asked. She took a bottle of nail polish from her pocket and reached for one of Elaine's hands. Elaine lifted her head, blinked at the bright red polish for a few seconds, then closed her eyes again.

"Neal?" said Cathryn. "Why don't you do that foot? He has one white foot."

"I don't want to."

"You don't want to? Well, finish the bear."

A woman in a drooping nightgown danced alone to the music. Another nearby rocked a doll, supporting it in the crook of her arm so the plastic face stared over her shoulder. She smiled placidly, as though pleased the baby wasn't crying. A rather youthful looking man dressed in work clothes had pulled a chair away from the others. He watched everyone in an alert way. I thought he might be a visitor, so I introduced myself. We talked about his wife, who is dying of cancer, and his farm over the western mountains, hunting with his son and grandson, his dogs, and an orchard of heirloom apple trees. I wondered who he was there to see, since no one seemed to be around him. Then the conversation started over.

5

A Friend in the Mid-Stage: Communication Toolkit

ACCEPT — DON'T ARGUE

A PERSON IN THE MID-STAGE of Alzheimer's disease trying to make sense of the world is like a pianist performing with three or four missing fingers. For a majority of people, honesty is essential in relationships. When accurate assimilation of information is no longer possible, the objective truth is not relevant. Honesty becomes more the higher aim of truthfully accepting the impediments of the disease than of sticking rigidly to facts. This is one of the main distinctions between the early and mid stages. Mild AD is not characterized by an almost constant state of disorientation. If statistics can be believed, a sizable percentage of normal-seeming people in late middle age are passing through the preclinical stage already. But after cognitive ability is compromised to a certain extent, the evidences of dementia cannot be mistaken except in a limited encounter. The consistent ability to think logically, react reasonably, speak clearly, and recognize familiar people and items is gone. No amount of persuasion, argument, or correction will alter this reality. While it may be instinctive to point out errors, sometimes in the misguided hope of jogging memory, the effort will likely lead to mutual frustration.

Friend: Oh, Aunt Martha! I'm happy to see you. It has been such a long time since you've visited.

You: I'm glad to see you, too. [*Instead of: I'm not Aunt Martha. Remember, your Aunt Martha passed away about twenty years ago. She was my grandmother. I've been told I look like her, but I'm Roberta.*]

Friend: Did you bring Stubby with you today?

You: No, Stubby isn't with me. [*Instead of: Who's Stubby? A dog? A short little boy?*]

Friend: Is Stubby here? Stubby loves to ride in the car. He never tries to jump into the front seat.

You: [*Repeating the last words*] Yes, he never jumps over the seat.

Friend: Did you bring Stubby?

You: No, he didn't come today. Do you miss Stubby? [*Instead of: I've told you twice I don't have a dog with me.*]

Friend: I love him. He's a good dog. Is he here? He doesn't like to be left outside.

You: No, but you love Stubby a lot, don't you? Here's a book with pictures of dogs. Let's look at it together.

ASK CLOSED QUESTIONS

Almost every guide on relationships advises asking open-ended questions to encourage free expression of ideas and feelings. To keep a conversation moving, we learn not to corral people with questions that restrict their response to yes or no. The opposite is true when talking with a friend in a more advanced stage of AD. As the disease disrupts the ability to form and articulate thoughts, being asked one of those encouraging "How do you feel? What do you think? What would you like?" questions can cause your friend to shut down rather than speak freely. Ask closed questions that supply an answer:

Instead of: "What do you want to do?"
Try: "Do you want to go for a walk?"

Instead of: "What do you need?"
Try: "Can I get you a sweater?"

Instead of: "How do you feel?"
Try: "You look sad. Are you missing somebody?"

Instead of: "What would you like to eat?"
Try: "Would you like a sandwich or tomato soup?"

Instead of: "How was your day?"
Try: "Are you tired from visiting your daughter?"

HANDLE HALLUCINATIONS GENTLY

Communications between people are anchored by the fact that we see and hear the same things, and our observations correspond to reality. AD can trigger hallucinations (perceptions) and delusions (beliefs) which seem completely real to the person experiencing them. It can feel strange to go along with the presence of people, animals, sounds, or threats that do not exist. Your friend, however, cannot help bringing you into these bizarre moments. They result from brain dysfunction and are not subject to reason or contradiction. Interact as best you can, adjusting to her interpretation of her surroundings. If the images bring about agitation, you might try ordering them to leave: "Shoo! Go away now. We need this room to ourselves."

You: I saw your grandson, Bobby, yesterday.

Friend: My grandson? I have five or six grandchildren. Did you say Bobby?

You: Yes, Bobby. The one who plays football at the high school with Coach Hall. They've got a fine team this year.

Friend: I don't know who they are. Who is that over by the window? I don't know half these people. They're strombers. I don't mean strombers! What word am I trying to say?

You: Are you trying to say strangers?

Friend: Don't you see those people? They're coming over here. Tell them to go away.

You: You people move on out of here. Go on. Why don't we sit somewhere else? They won't follow us. [*Pausing between separate topics* [21]] Bobby is playing football this year.

Friend: Bobby? Who's Bobby? Is he your son?

You: [*Continuing to speak calmly—not increasing the volume of your voice, as though your friend might be losing his hearing instead of his mind*] No, I saw your grandson, Bobby.

Friend: I don't know their names. I don't know.

You: [*Shifting to the distant past*] Did you ever play football, yourself?

Friend: I played football for Hardwood High School. We won the championship my last year.

You: I never knew that.

Friend: It was a game to remember. That thirty-yard touchdown happened in the last seconds. It was one of the happiest days of my life.

You: What position did you play?

Friend: I was a running back. Did I ever tell you about my thirty-yard touchdown?

BEAR WITH REPETITIVENESS

Adelle (from chapter 1) is unusual, having stayed in the early stage longer than most with AD, probably due to her participation in a clinical trial. She can drive safely, care for her personal needs, socialize, and stay at home alone. She engages in critical thinking and functions appropriately for the most part as a wife and grandmother. Her constant repetitiveness, however, indicates an ominous swing toward more serious incapacity.

A person with mid-stage AD can sometimes arrange words into sentences, although language abilities markedly decline as the disease goes on. She may be unaware of having spoken, and her grasp of her surroundings and circumstances is tenuous. When the hippocampus no longer functions, the recollection of what has just been said, done, or experienced is gone in a matter of minutes. One conversation can seem like multiple rehearsals for a short play scene in which the same animated lines are delivered again and again.

In mid-stage AD, the recollection of what has just been said, done, or experienced is often gone in a matter of minutes.

The kindest response is to reply as though hearing for the first time the repeated stories and questions. Regrettably, few of us are so patient. By mid-stage, a reminder that you've already been told something (see page thirty-six) will not be effective. Try pairing the visit with an activity you can do simultaneously (needlepoint, snapping beans, brushing a long-haired dog, polishing shoes, reorganizing a toolbox or drawer—anything that doesn't require your full concentration and quietly takes place in one room or area). Here is an example:

You: Winfred, do you mind if I bring down my laundry to fold while we talk?

Friend: Not at all. You go right ahead.

You: Thanks. I'm so far behind, and the children are coming this weekend.

Friend: The most upsetting thing has happened to me. I don't know what to do. We're moving next month! Ernest told me about it this morning. I'd rather walk over hot coals than pack. What will we do with Baby Cat?

You: Where are you going? [*Instead of: Don't be silly. You've lived in the house next door for the past twenty years. Ernie just repaired the back deck and bought a new grill.*]

Friend: We're moving to Texas.

You: I've lived in a lot of places, never Texas. That's a long way away.

Friend: Yes, it is. My goodness, how time flies. Did I mention that Ernest and I are moving soon? He told me about it this morning over the scrambled eggs. Just waved his fork in the air and said, "Winnie, start packing!"

You: You're going to Texas, right? Have you been there before?

Friend: Ernest is going to Longhorn College. I never thought we'd move. I don't want to leave this place. I'm so upset.

You: [*Responding to the emotion*] I can tell you're upset. But you know how men are—always making big plans. He'll probably change his mind.

Friend: Yes, I do know about men. Can't live with them, and can't live without them. I should have left Ernest when he bought that leaky old houseboat. Do you know he told me this morning we have to move again?

REVISIT THE PAST

Memories of past relationships, jobs, and homes may be stored in the mind like dusty photo albums on shelves, albeit in a diffuse, far less systematic way. If you've ever climbed into the dimness of an attic and flicked on the light to read faded letters or look at school notebooks and term papers, then you know the waves of nostalgia revisiting those times can bring. Your friend may believe she is living decades earlier and sometimes can talk about that part of her life. The capacity for short term memory is affected by AD first, long-term memories not until later in the disease. Be where she is in the moment, understanding that you need to go along into her mind's "attic" to help her find and use the words that have meaning.

Friend: [*In her own family room*] I want to go home.

You: Are you tired of being here? Maybe you're cold. Let me get your afghan for you. [*Asking to go home can be a way of expressing physical discomfort.*]

Friend: I want to go home now.

You: We'll go after a while. Tell me about your home.

Friend: It's the brick house on East Madison where Helen and I live. Have you seen Helen? Is she at the school where she teaches?

You: Yes, I think probably she is. [*Instead of: Are you talking about your sister?*

Helen lives in Nebraska with Ida May now. She won't be coming back to visit until Christmas, and she hasn't taught school since the early nineties.]

Friend: I need to call Helen. Can you get me her number at work? I need to call her. She could come and get me.

You: You'd like to talk with Helen?

Friend: It's getting late, and I need to go home! What's wrong with you?

You: Why don't we call her when she's not working? Don't worry, I know you want to go home. Tell me about Helen. I never met her.

Friend: Well, Helen's very smart, but poor thing, she can barely see past her own nose. She was so very glad to get glasses a few years ago. The children at school love her. Can you call her for me?

OVERLOOK PARANOIA

Paranoia develops in about one-third of AD patients and must be understood as a symptom of the disease, nothing more. Suspicions and accusations do not merit upset or grave acknowledgment on your part. Dispassionately respond to the underlying emotion of anger or frustration and attempt to redirect your friend's attention.

Friend: Where is my pearl necklace?

You: I don't know. I haven't seen it.

Friend: Don't tell me that. You have. You took it!

You: You're worried about the necklace, aren't you? [*Instead of: I absolutely did not. How can you say that?*]

Friend: Yes, I am. My Uncle Archie brought that necklace back from the Caribbean for my grandmother, and you need to give it back.

You: Your Grandmother Josie? Did she give it to you a long time ago?

Friend: She gave it to me, and she's going to be hurt if I'm not wearing it next time she comes to the house.

You: I'll help you look for it. We can find it by then. [*Reassure, then change the focus of the conversation to a pleasant event that happened repeatedly in the past.*] I can almost see your Grandmother Josie sitting on the porch swing with Miss Sassy, that big orange cat nobody else could touch.

Friend: Miss Sassy lived to be twenty-three years old and never liked anybody much. I remember when she got her head caught in the chicken coop. All the hens were running around flapping their wings, and she was yowling.

REACT CALMLY TO AGGRESSION

Irrational, aggressive behavior is alarming, especially when it seems to come out of the blue. Patients with AD may go through periods of agitation in which they are predisposed to verbal outbursts and, less frequently, physical aggression. It may be triggered by an invasion of personal space, pain or discomfort, delusional thinking, and increased frustration. If a person no longer remembers how to work a toaster or put on a jacket, you can imagine how constant her struggle must be to interpret the barrage of stimuli we face in a given day. For most of us, anger is a common defense against threat. With AD, predicting what will be perceived as a threat can be difficult. The moves we unthinkingly make to enhance communication may appear confrontational when separated from the related words. Consider the following:

Words: "Julia is leaving to work with the Peace Corps. I'm worried. If I could hold onto her for one more year, I'd feel better."

Gesture: Outstretched, closed hands

Words: "And when Jenn opened the gate, Buck galloped right at me. I didn't think he'd stop, but I stood my ground and yelled 'Whoa!'"

Gesture: Open hands, thrust in the direction of the listener

Making sense of such actions requires instant comprehension and integration of the verbal context, a complex encoding process most of us take for granted. By the mid-stage, many AD patients have lost the ability to understand ambiguity. A fist means only one thing, and it's not passionate concern for a grown child. Try to refrain from movements which could appear hostile.

Keep sentences short and simple. "Let's go to your room" will be less annoying than "Do you want to go back to your own room now? It's noisy in this recreation room. I wish they had a common area that didn't have a television blaring, don't you? Oh dear, here comes the arts and crafts group. I'll hold your arm to steady you." Also, be alert to your friend's body language. People who are tired and irritated sometimes do not like to talk or be touched, whether they have dementia or not. They would rather be left alone.

If aggressive behavior has been observed in the past, a caregiver should stay closeby to intervene at the first sign of escalating emotion. In case of a flare-up, keep calm. Don't react with your own anger. Remind yourself that your friend cannot control her emotions, but you can yours. Step away to give her space and a few minutes to unwind, a prudent reaction throughout life to any person who is about to fly off the handle. Think about what happened just before the reaction, because this event likely contributed to it. In a conciliatory tone, reassure your friend you will remedy the problem: "Wait a minute, I'll [*take the puzzle away, turn the radio off, move over to the other chair, get Belinda to come back, put Puff outside, help you find your glasses*]. Everything is okay."

> *Remind yourself that your friend cannot control her emotions, but you can yours.*

FIT THE PIECES TOGETHER

Problems with word retrieval may make formulating a single sentence difficult and organizing thoughts impossible. Speculate as best you can about what your friend is trying to say and supply the missing words. As mentioned before, be sensitive to nonverbal signals indicating appreciation for help and not increased frustration. If speech has regressed to a mixed salad of words, respond to the nonverbal dimension and forego any effort to impose logic on what you are hearing.[22] Chapter 12 shows how to handle this kind of dialogue. Here is an example of how you might successfully fit together fragments arising from a partially intact recollection:

You: You've been on a long trip, Bob.

Friend: Long trip, long trip.

You: A lot of miles in the car.

Friend: Yes. I didn't…didn't…. Gone. The thought's gone.

You: Didn't do the driving?

Friend: Yes, didn't do the driving.

You: Rita drove the whole time, then.

Friend: That's right. Right.

You: You saw your son and his family.

Friend: That's right. It was good. Good.

You: You've done a lot of traveling over the years, haven't you, Bob?

Friend: Yes, that's right.

You: Here's a photo album of the trip you and Rita took for your honeymoon. Look, here's Rita on the coastline at Big Sur. That was a long time ago.

Friend: Beautiful Rita. I miss Rita. I miss her very much.

You: I'll bet you do. I miss Greg. [*Instead of: "Wait, Bob. Rita's right here in this room. The two of you just went to Connecticut together." The present-day Rita may look completely different from the Rita of forty years earlier, the period of life your friend remembers. He may recognize photos of a younger Rita but not very often the one who now takes care of him.*]

ENSURE A SECURE SITUATION

In the mid-stage, an Alzheimer's patient may resist separation from her caregiver, upon whom she now relies for almost everything. The caregiver would no doubt welcome a break, but before taking on the role of temporary caregiver yourself, ask whether your friend might become excessively anxious with her usual caregiver gone. If so, the caregiver could remain in the vicinity, taking more of a psychological time-out than a physical one.

The need for constant connection with the caregiver varies from person to person. Elaine, mentioned in the previous chapter, enjoyed the company of others well into the late stage of the disease. College students "adopted" her and took her out for lunch and short trips around the city. In contrast, Joe, formerly an army colonel accustomed to barking orders, would not have appreciated such excursions, even with two pretty young women. Joe had lacked Elaine's gregarious nature throughout life, and this tendency toward social introversion grew more pronounced in the course of dementia. During one period of his illness, he became agitated and angry when he was not in his wife's presence. It would have been unwise then for a friend to have taken Joe away in the car, assuming she could drive safely while dealing with his unpredictable, potentially volatile reaction to a change in environment. Pay attention to your friend's body language and emotional state, looking for confirmation of her ease and feeling of safety.

6

Help When Caregiving Gets Harder

RECOGNIZE THE DIFFERENCES

A CAREGIVER, LYNDA, DESCRIBES HOW HER LIFE has changed over a five-year period as her husband went from being an active retired college professor, involved in starting teacher education programs in developing countries, to being unable to read a newspaper. "He went all over the world until he had his own world narrowed down," she says. "I recognize the look of confusion: *What day is it? Who am I? Where are we?* It's just... it's just...." She deliberates a few moments to find the right word. "It's just sad. Because the person you knew isn't there any more. I do everything now. *All* of it. I do absolutely everything. I can tell him, 'Come in here and help me fix breakfast. Here, why don't you help me butter the toast?' And he stands there with that knife in his hand. I have to put the butter right under his nose."

Imagine Lynda saying those exact words to a friend. The friend responds, "I know what you mean. Jim gets himself a beer and kicks back on the couch with the TV remote while I'm trying to fix dinner every night. I didn't mind so much before he retired. He was on his feet from nine to five at the paint store, but now? He sits around. When I ask for help, he gives me this blank look and says, 'With what?' like I need to spell it out. Like he's a little kid."

Any caregiver would be tempted to say without a hint of sarcasm, "You're lucky."

Lynda had adopted a new lens through which to view her situation, and her philosophy can serve as a guide for friendships. "I'm trying to think of this as a time when I am living a different life," she says. "I have so many years to live. These years are going to be this way. I'm in love with my husband, and, yes, the circumstances have changed. I'm trying to find a different approach to that love."

A different approach to friendship during this period could mean an effort to be more sensitive than before and to keep in mind the severity of your friend's problems. Here is how the same snippet of conversation might then play out:

Friend: And he stands there with that knife in his hand, looking at me. I have to put the butter right under his nose. He can't butter toast anymore.

You: I listen to you, and I think my predicament with Jim isn't so bad. I've been angry with him for lying on the sofa like a beached whale while I cook dinner. Last night I told him he's spoiled and lazy. He slammed his beer down and went straight to Jessie and Reva's house. But at least he knows what I'm complaining about. You can't hold it against Harry for not helping.

Friend: Harry and I never fought much. We had looked forward our whole married life to retirement. We were going to build a house at the lake. We'd been planning it since we were in our twenties, but it wasn't meant to be. Were you and Jim able to talk later?

You: I can't talk to him anymore. I don't know how things got so tense. We're worried about money, and neither of us wants to go back to work.

Friend: I'm not in your shoes, but I understand what not having any help around the house is like.

You: I know you do. Maybe better than anyone else.

FOCUS ON FEELINGS

Caregiving is lonely. It leads to anger at the person with Alzheimer's disease for being sick and uncooperative. It leads to anger at yourself for being impatient, for being unable to work out the never-ending stream of problems, and for not having done more before the disease took away the chance. It leads to anxiety over the cost of professional services or assisted living and the lack, sometimes, of tenable alternatives. Many caregivers are grieving. Unlike the grief following death, with a memorial service, an outpouring of sympathy, a mourning period, and in time a new beginning, it goes on for up to two decades in the incremental loss, trait by trait, of a beloved person and a relationship in which a lifetime may have been invested.

You may not ever have to witness a loved one labor along with a failing brain or yourself take care of an adult who has forgotten how to care for himself, but we've all felt sadness, stress, fear, fatigue, uncertainty, loneliness, anger, and boredom. Give your friend a place to speak freely, realizing you share the range of these emotions for other reasons. As indicated in the previous example, though, acknowledge the differences in what brought about your strong feelings and qualify any comparisons: "I know this isn't the same as what you're going through, but I lost half my retirement in the financial crisis. I can't make up for it, and I'm worried, too, about running out of money." A caregiver may face simultaneously a similar loss of security and the responsibility of supporting a parent or spouse who requires skilled full-time care for a period of years.

When the caregiver needs to talk, don't problem solve or moralize. Reflect emotion and ask nonintrusive questions that show interest and concern. It will be enough. Consider the following two dialogues. Which would you find more helpful?

The Opinionated Friend

Friend: I had a contract fall through at work yesterday. I was depending on it for Jay's tuition. When I got home, I heard Meg's father yelling as soon as I opened the door: "Don't turn off the light switches! I can turn off fifty light switches!" I walked right back out.

You: You shouldn't have left. Meg was probably mad at both of you then. Why don't you find a nursing home for him? They know how to handle old people.

Friend: Meg quit her job to look after her father. We've got two kids in college. Do you know how much nursing homes cost? The only one nearby is ninety thousand dollars a year. Bill didn't have long-term care insurance. His house is a wreck. It won't sell without work, and he doesn't qualify for Medicaid.

You: Why don't you hire someone to help her? That's what I'd do.

Friend: Because like I said, we don't have the money. We can't afford to hire someone for the night if we want to go out, and it's hard to find the right person. Most of the agencies send out women. When he's mad, he shouts every word he ever heard in the Marines. He doesn't want a strange woman helping him dress if he needs to change clothes. He's usually quiet with Meg, even if he doesn't know he's her father anymore.

You: Why don't you get some kind of medication to make him calm? My doctor would prescribe it. They have those drugs. My dog had to be put on an antidepressant for separation anxiety, and it works really well. He used to bark and claw the paint off the doors for hours. It drove everybody crazy, so I know how you feel.

Friend: My father-in-law is already on an antidepressant. He's on sleeping pills and a lot of other things we can't get him to take, from three different doctors. He's eighty-seven. Why is he still around, anyway? I don't think I want to be here at eighty-seven.

You: Think about what you're saying. You sound like Kevorkian. I wish my dad were still alive. He died when I was ten.

The Compassionate Friend

Friend: I had a contract fall through at work yesterday. I don't know what I'll do for Jay's tuition. When I got home, I could hear Meg's father yelling some nonsense about light switches. She was mad at me for leaving. I can't do anything right except pay the bills. I know she's got her hands full, but I do, too.

You: How long has your father-in-law been this way?

Friend: For about eight months. When he first moved in with us, he couldn't do much, but he seemed content.

You: Does your wife stay home with him?

Friend: Every single day. She quit her job because she wanted to take care of him. We never go out anymore. It wasn't as hard when we could leave him alone for a few hours or take him with us. His doctor says he could go on for years. No problems with his heart or anything. He's strong for eighty-seven.

You: What was he like before he got Alzheimer's?

Friend: Great sense of humor, patient. He never raised his voice. He started taking Jay fishing with him as soon as we'd let him go. Jay spent a lot of time with his granddad on the boat. Those were good summers. He made beautiful furniture, too. For Meg's fortieth birthday, he made her a china cabinet with inlays and leaded glass. He and Meg were always close.

You: He sounds like my father. He died when I was ten. It must be tough for the whole family, especially Meg.

Friend: Her father wasn't loud and paranoid at first. It's a phase of dementia with some people, and it will probably get better in time. I wish we could hire outside help, but we're too strapped for cash.

You: Paying college tuition for two kids has got to make it worse.

Friend: I don't know how we'll afford everything. I wasn't prepared for this expense. We've always had two incomes in the past.

You: I don't know what I'd do, but is there a support group in town? There must be other people who are going through this, and they might know some options you haven't thought about. I could check into it for you.

DO LISTEN, DON'T ADVISE

For a caregiver, responding to unwelcome advice is like dodging a misguided motorist on a one-way street. No matter how sincere your concern or how right you are in your observations, a person outside a relationship cannot fully appreciate the physical and emotional complexity of the problems, particularly in a situation like AD. Try to refrain from giving advice unless you are asked for it, and then offer ideas only after listening carefully.

Friend: I'm so tired. John wanders around every night. I was up twice after midnight. At around three, he had pulled the sheets and covers off his bed. I made bacon and eggs this morning, because he seems to get along better when he has a good breakfast. He hardly ate any. By the time I talked him into going to the adult center, it was eleven o'clock.

You: I'm worried about you, Ellen. How are you taking care of yourself? [*Instead of: Why don't you put a lock on the guest room where he sleeps and wear earplugs?*]

Friend: Take care of myself? When? More and more lately, he says "I want Ellen!" like I'm not myself. He has no clue I'm his wife. I'm just that old curly-haired lady who makes him mad.

You: I had no idea what you were dealing with.

Friend: Last week his sister criticized me for selling his car. She said I should have kept it, so he could drive around the nice quiet neighborhood and feel independent every now and then. Not a concern for her. She won't be riding a bicycle or walking her dog while he enjoys this independence in several thousand pounds of gasoline-powered steel. What if he made it to the freeway?

You: Has his sister spent a week or two with him lately?

Friend: She doesn't want to stay with him. She wants to be several hundred miles away, telling me what to do.

JUDGE NOT...

A quick ride on a high horse often begins with the phrase, "I would never [*say, act like, or do*] that!" Most of us have been guilty of mentally projecting ourselves into someone else's life and speculating about how much better we would manage our own emotions. Assume the caregiver is doing the best he can under trying circumstances, many of which are not plainly evident, and respond with empathy to any confessions of breakdown or rancor, as long as the angry reactions are infrequent and nonviolent. Mistreatment or potential abuse is a different issue. A supportive attitude is particularly important when the caregiver is contemplating residential care for his loved one. In these examples, an empathetic response is appropriate:

Friend: I promised my parents I would never put them in a nursing home, but I don't know anymore. I can't watch my dad every minute. He dropped his cigarette on the floor and walked away. I found it smoldering. What if the house had caught fire?

You: That's a big decision. When you made the promise, you didn't know it would turn out this way. I'll bet your father wouldn't have let you promise if he had known, either. You can love and support him wherever he is. [*Instead of: I wouldn't put either of my parents in an institution. They took care of me, and I'll take care of them no matter what. Why are you letting him smoke? Throw away the cigarettes. Then you won't have to worry about that.*]

Friend: I shouted at my mother this afternoon. She asked me for the hundredth time where her mother was, and I lost it. My daughter dropped a glass pitcher of tea on the stone floor, and it shattered everywhere. I hollered at Mom to get out of the way. Only, I used awful words. She looked so hurt.

You: Don't be hard on yourself. Everybody loses control once in a while. You should have heard what I said when Bud spilled a bucket of white paint on the carpet. Did your mom remember it later? [*Instead of: Well, you really shouldn't have yelled at her. She can't help what she says, can she?*]

The following example shows when to be concerned the problem is more than an occasional outburst which will be quickly forgotten by the person with dementia:

Friend: I'm scared of my own temper lately. I can't believe how furious I am at my mother. When she's dripping around the house in that horrible maroon bathrobe, slamming cabinets and doors and looking like if she had a gun, she'd shoot me, I want to shake her! I'm trying my best. I don't know where she finds the energy to be so obnoxious. And she's gotten so fragile in the past year, her skin is like tissue paper. I barely grabbed her arm the other day, and she has a huge bruise. I didn't mean to hurt her. I was upset. I love her, but I don't know how to go on like this.

You: I've been worried that taking care of your mother is getting too stressful. I'll call the Alzheimer's Association.* They'll know how to help. There may be support in the community. I can sit with your mom while you meet with them.

EASE AWAY EMBARRASSMENT

Although a person in the middle stage can appear normal, the illusion is quickly lost when his composure, no longer underpinned by a sense of social mores or personal responsibility, gives way at an inopportune moment. Loss of inhibition and inappropriate sexual behaviors sometimes crop up in mid-stage, and a sudden breach of control in this area is particularly unsettling.

A caregiver was grocery shopping one morning with her husband in tow. Before she could intervene, he unzipped his trousers, which fell to the floor. A man took his wife for a rare outing to a restaurant, and she rushed inside and threw her arms around the startled hostess, as

*Alzheimer's Association contact information:
www.alz.org / 1-800-272-3900 / info@alz.org

though she had just met a long lost friend. Another caregiver reported that her father made lewd gestures and gibes to young women, even his own granddaughters. People in public are more inclined to gape or stare in consternation than conclude charitably there must be a reasonable explanation, which is hard for a caregiver caught unexpectedly in the limelight. Alzheimer's disease can be an invisible illness, providing casual onlookers no clue anything is really wrong. Briefly explain to them that there is a medical cause for the incident, if need be, and help your friends move on.

UNDERSTAND THE LOSS

I spent an afternoon in an artist's studio in North Carolina, left vacant for several years. Sunlight streamed through tall windows, and the faint smell of turpentine still lingered. Paintings lined the walls. Her presence was so vivid in the bold lines and colors, I could almost see her sitting at a large wooden easel, creating works displayed in some of the nation's most prestigious galleries. The easel stood off to one side, as though she might return at any moment to finish the drawing pinned to it. With a tightly controlled face, her husband spoke about the long marriage the two had shared, a marriage that had eluded the common pitfalls of tedium and detachment. He confessed his dread at finding her one day, collapsed in a nearby field, lost and confused. Eventually her dementia made it impossible for him to care for her alone. He visits her daily in the nursing home where she lives now, unable to respond anymore to art. She recognizes him and repeats "I love you" back to him. They hug and kiss.

"She isn't lost to me yet. People tell me over and over again I've done the right thing, not to feel guilty. They see I'm suffering, but what am I suffering?" he asked, clearly disquieted at having been misunderstood by his friends. "I am suffering the loss *she* is suffering," he said, stressing each word, so I would not miss the point, too. The deepest part of his sadness was not his own deprivation or fear of wrongdoing but rather the sorrow he felt on his wife's behalf for the losses she could no longer comprehend.

The feelings of grief are similar among people—despondency, heartache, loneliness, fear. But the relationship, whether between child and parent, life partners, best friends or siblings, is as unique as the two

Don't assume you understand; let your friend tell his story.

people who became intimate within its framework of circumstances. Don't assume you understand; let your friend tell his story. Caregivers, despite the tremendous demands, often feel lovingly attached to the person with dementia. "We've been married for fifty-seven years," said another caregiver of his wife. "Whether she knows me or not, she sleeps right beside me at night with her arm around me. I'm her security."

"You're a good man," I told him. We were having lunch together, and he'd described how much he loves his wife, how protective he is of her, given her vulnerable state.

"She's a good woman," he replied.

THINK THROUGH

Herman, a caregiver who stoically accepted his wife's diagnosis of AD, was determined to give her as many years of happiness after retirement as he could. She had raised his children from a previous marriage and supported him in his climb to a top position in the field of school administration. He didn't grieve over her illness. He considered himself privileged to care for her and found meaning, he said, in the challenge to become a stronger, better person in response to her dementia. However, during trying moments, he remembered the Biblical adage "This too shall pass." *It will get better,* he told himself, realizing deep down the falseness of the hope.

Known as an even-tempered negotiator, Herman was adept at using wit and humor to lead people. In the end, he held the purse strings of a billion dollar education budget. He had handled deftly the maelstrom of emotion and competing motivations provoked by such a large sum of money, but he was brought to a state of plain fear by his frail wife in mid-stage AD. *What will happen tomorrow,* he wondered, *next week, next year? What will I do? How will I take care of her?* In spite of these questions, he projected a tough unshakable front for his family. One daughter, calling her father's bluff, gently helped him confront the worries that badgered him. "Okay," she'd say, "but what if it doesn't get better? The next time she falls, and you can't get her up, what can you do?" This approach was better for Herman than either scoffing at or accepting his optimistic facade.

Alternatives are empowering but hard to generate when anxiety is in full throttle. In managing a tide of unpredictable behaviors and abilities, caregivers live on the brink of crisis. While refraining from peremptory advice-giving, help your friend calmly think through the problems he anticipates:

- "Should we make a list to post beside the phone of neighbors and relatives you can contact in an emergency, or program the numbers into your cell phone?"

- "Do you need a sounding board for your financial options? I can listen in confidence."

- "If he does wander away, what will you do? Is he registered with Safe Return?* Let's decide how to respond now, before it happens."

- "What would be the advantages of moving your mother into your home? Try to imagine making that choice. Are you more relieved or concerned when you picture her living with your family?"

---

*MedicAlert + Safe Return® is a nationwide emergency response service in which dementia patients are enrolled. An engraved identification bracelet or pendant can be purchased for both the patient and the caregiver to wear. The jewelry provides a toll-free number, monitored 24/7. For information, contact the Alzheimer's Association (800-272-3900 or info@alz.org).

PART THREE

The Last Years

7

Velma's Story

*For her last birthday, we took three kinds of ice cream to my
grandmother's room. And, of course, every patient who saw us
was right there! We scooped twenty-five or thirty ice cream cones
with sprinkles. My daughter, Kate, was learning how to hold
her cone, so my mom and I got them up on the bed together
and covered them with sheets and towels. They laughed their
heads off because ice cream and sprinkles were everywhere. The
ice cream would fall off my grandmother's cone, and she would
pick it up and say to Kate, "I'm not doing much better than you
are!" Then Kate would knock the ice cream off her own cone
and laugh.*

*It was one of my most precious memories. It was such a gift. It
was good just to be there in a moment when you didn't have to
do it right.*

— Teresa

Teresa's Grandmother Velma grew up as the oldest child
of sharecroppers on an Arkansas cotton farm. She wore clothing
made of flour sacks. At age five, only three years older than Kate
on the afternoon they spent giggling and dripping with ice cream,

she was sent alone down the rows of cotton with a stick to flush out poisonous snakes before her father worked the fields—a father himself born to an unwed girl in a shotgun shack with quilts pinned shamefully over the windows and his grandfather standing guard at the front door with a gun. Velma left home, as might be expected, with emotional problems that greatly complicated her adult relationships. In the last year of her life, Alzheimer's disease had stripped away her phobias and compulsions, along with the awareness of who she was and had been. It happened almost methodically, Teresa said, "like layers being peeled off of an onion."

Teresa and I talked about her grandmother one morning in the corner of a coffee shop crammed with tables and too many people. A high ceiling and the clash of voices made it seem more like a theater lobby at intermission. Even in the commotion, Teresa's eyes filled with tears, not the urgent tears of fresh grief but the ones that quietly slip out when we wade very far into the memories of someone loved and lost. She brushed them from her face, almost in annoyance. I sensed in her immediacy and passion a love for Velma that neither dementia nor death had altered.

Her stories, spanning decades, were lively and close to the surface. She remembers being served a dinner of lime Jell-O mixed with Russian salad dressing. Velma had mild dementia then, and Teresa, at the height of adolescence, had laughed helplessly at the chopped pickles jiggling in muddy brown gelatin, despite her father's reproachful kicks under the table. One afternoon she awoke from a nap and was startled to find herself in an encampment of teddy bears. Giving rein to her quirky sense of fun, Velma had gathered up the bears and tucked them around Teresa, careful not to disturb her sleep.

To the day she died, her grandmother knew her, which is seldom the case. By the time Alzheimer's reaches the final stage, the cerebral hemispheres, in youth plump and packed within the skull like the flesh of perfectly ripened fruit, have shriveled and pulled inward. For Teresa's grandmother to have recognized and said goodbye to her family at the end was highly unusual.

More often, death from advanced Alzheimer's (instead of a complication) comes after a person has lost virtually everything.[23] A woman I met when beginning my research several years ago has gone from mid-stage AD, chattering and exploring her surroundings with apparent interest in the constant newness of it all, to lying curled, barely moving, in a hospice bed. Occasionally she mutters, and she can swallow. Soon these reflexes will be gone, too.

Dementia cannot be compared easily to other organ-specific maladies because of the brain's resiliency and intricate control of every bodily function. What remains of the brain in mid-to-late AD is nonetheless complex, bringing the potential for random behavior and differences between people with similar patterns of damage. One man with younger-onset AD went steadily along in the mid-stage for more than a decade, before he became so incapacitated his wife arranged placement for him in a nursing home. Leaving their house with clothing and toiletries packed, he shuffled out to the car and insisted, as he always had, on opening her door in a gesture of courtliness. She thanked him, then jumped out and sprinted around the back fender to help him with his own door. The same man was led in handcuffs from the noisy, chaotic facility by the police a few weeks later for having reportedly cornered himself behind a barricade of furniture in what may have been, on an intuitive level, a sensible response to a setup that probably seemed more to him like past years in Vietnam than a new place to live.

UNLIKE MOST PEOPLE in the late stage of AD, Velma kept her speech, putting words purposively together, until just before death and was thus able to change within her own mind some of the more troubled parts of her past. Settled into the confines of a nursing home after staying alone during a precarious middle phase, she redid her daughter's wedding. Teresa's mother, Ruth, had married the son of a sharecropper, and her failure to secure a higher social rank through one of the more readily available means provoked Velma's caustic disapproval. Her sole contribution to the bridal festivities had been a demand that her daughter choose a more expensive china pattern. Fifty years later, Velma stepped into her role as mother of the bride. She was full of plans. Teresa would be a bridesmaid, and she'd wear a blue and burgundy dress. Kate would be the flower girl. They would carry lilies. Ruth, who had worn a wedding dress sewn by an aunt and posted the invitation in a few local church bulletins, charitably agreed. "Sure, Mom," she'd say, with superhuman patience, "I think a Saturday in May would be nice. Yes, let's serve punch." Until at last, the redemption was complete. Velma had done it the way she should have and perhaps at the time had wanted deep down, but of greater importance, she had found a way of apologizing.

Although dementia is grievously unfair, there was a hint of recompense in Velma's cognitive losses. Determined to wrest something more from life than an endless strand of days in a field, she finished high school with honors and established herself as a beautician. She washed, fixed, colored, and curled away the stigma of having grown up poor. Yet she was powerless to remedy her deep insecurity. Velma spent most of her life afraid. As the disease escalated, so did the paranoia which had distorted her thinking since childhood. For a particularly taxing period of months, she would call Teresa every half hour or so, day and night, crying that she was being beaten, the nurses hated her, people were after her. She concocted elaborate schemes for escape from the nursing home and sordid stories about Teresa's father. Teresa, dealing then with Kate's passage from infancy to toddlerhood, wisely stopped answering the phone. In the long run, those neural pathways were cleared away, and Velma was left with fragments of memories distilled from the complications of anger and shame. As she talked freely about her past for the first time, Teresa and Ruth began to fit the stories together like fragments of broken china, reassembling a family history they had never known.

Throughout adult life, Velma had compensated for her sense of inadequacy with notions of racial superiority, regrettably not an uncommon gambit. As her dementia worsened, the dyke of civility within her personality crumbled, and her unrestrained racial slurs would stop traffic, Teresa said. By the late stage, Velma had forgotten not only the vocabulary but the reasons for her discrimination. People were just people, and ethnicity no longer mattered. Her last roommate was an African American woman, for whom Velma cared as lovingly as she would have her own mother, laying out her gown at night and checking to make sure her false teeth had been put in a glass of water.

Alzheimer's disease does not generally inspire a sense of peace and acceptance of other people. Sadly, the opposite is often true. A woman who had been coping reasonably well with memory loss awoke from the anesthesia for surgery to repair a broken hip cursing like a drunken sailor. She was never the same again. "It was a night and day difference," her daughter, Jenny, recalled. "Oh, my goodness, she was nasty! She called my father every name in the book and was suspicious of people. It was terrible. She'd spit on the nurses; she would hiss. You had to worry she'd try to harm you. Unfortunately that was an overriding characteristic of her dementia until she quit communicating." [24]

It didn't change her husband's love. Any marriage therapist who has had a session spiral into a screaming match will tell you embedded resentments are hard to undo. But in the absence of deliberate hurt or betrayal, so is passionately held affection. When Jenny's mother forgot how to swallow, her father would sit by the bed, massaging morsels of food down her throat. He helped her to live months longer than doctors believed she could.

Late stage Alzheimer's disease returns a person to a state in many ways like infancy—only, though, in lost abilities. Even at the very end, when body and mind have almost shut down, there is an adult present with a life history of accomplishments a disease cannot take away. Velma's family recognized her unchanged right to be treated with dignity. Ruth kept her in clean clothes and set her hair weekly. Velma may not have recognized her daughter or cared any more about a hairstyle so crucial to her self-image at the height of life that she had trained herself to sleep sitting straight up to preserve it. She did realize she was being given considerable assistance. In a newly acquired state of humbleness, she said "thank you" over and over, stunning Ruth, who had long lived under the steady drumbeat of her mother's criticism. Nothing Ruth did was ever enough, until Velma lost both her trait of discontent and control of her bladder. "You didn't do this for me. You've disappointed me! You could have been so much more. Your husband isn't good enough. Your children don't act right. I expected you to turn out better" became, as Ruth folded freshly laundered clothes and combed Velma's hair, "Oh, thank you. Thank you so much for what you do for me. Thank you for caring so well." Teresa said her grandmother's words were like an axe, chipping away at a backlog of hurts.

Ruth's intimate care of her mother was difficult in part because the laundry smelled so awful. Everything reeked of urine, and the stench permeated her car and her own clothing, her own hair. The palpable memory of it persisted after Velma died. One dubious mercy of Alzheimer's disease by the end stage, when incontinence invariably poses a problem, is that it destroys the sense of smell. The fragile nerves of the olfactory bulb fall to the disease early on. One caregiver said her husband's physician blindfolded him after he complained of memory loss and checked his ability to distinguish between common scents, like lemon, gasoline, smoke, and vanilla. He couldn't identify any of them. So Velma, whose life was spent helping women show a well-coiffed front to the public, was not aware she had fallen so far into helplessness. Ruth's realization that her mother could no longer keep herself clean enabled her to begin emotionally letting go of the relationship. She knew her mother would never get better, but much worse.

Alzheimer's disease is relentless, claiming regions of the brain like a steadily advancing army with crosshairs aimed first at the most sophisticated targets: the ability to learn and reason, the sense of direction, abstract and sequential thinking, and the attachment of emotion to reality. Finally it takes anything that is left. Velma's loss of skills began to coincide with her great granddaughter's acquisition of them. Kate, with only the most rudimentary psychological needs—kindness, predictability, attention—and no storehouse of past hurts and expectations, accepted her great grandmother's mistakes and regressions as a matter of inconsequential fact. Kate wasn't grieved that Velma could not think of words, understand the difference between fact and fantasy, or dress and bathe herself. Kate couldn't do those things either. With a small child's incomprehension of time except as related to the necessities of food, play and sleep, Kate lived in the moment with Velma, and theirs was a simple, undemanding love. When she was learning to write, Kate composed a letter which summed it up: "Grandma Velma, God loves you. You are fun. I love you. Love, Kate K."

DISTRACTED AND PULLED IN MANY DIRECTIONS, mired in irksome life circumstances, and sometimes just plain tired and stressed out, we adults find it hard to downshift to a gear in which only what is immediately happening matters, and the energy and good intentions we invest will be instantly forgotten. A daughter, Sarah, lives several hundred miles from her mother, stricken by Alzheimer's disease in her mid-seventies. Sarah has a busy life with her own family, but she dearly loves her mother and can hardly speak of her without tears. Regardless of these tender feelings, she described her frustration on one occasion with her mother's bewilderment in the bathroom. "I had her standing in front of the toilet, and she had no idea what to do. I kept saying, 'Please, please, sit down!' I tried to explain. She was confused and kept grabbing at my hands and shaking my shoulders." Her voice was tinged with the upset of having had a chunk of time fall away in trying to bring about something so basic.

Sarah's mother, unlike Velma, had gone from being the "wise owl" of the family, the one to whom people had always turned for advice and unconditional love, to someone who would lose in the end even her characteristic smile. Her affliction with Alzheimer's disease was particularly cruel. Perceptive enough to know she was failing in a dreadful way, she could not comprehend why. Throughout a Christmas holiday, years into the disease, she sat around and cried disconsolately. One of her granddaughters climbed in her lap and asked, "Gramma, what's wrong?"

"I don't know. I don't know," she replied, hugging the child.

While Sarah's mother felt the best parts of herself draining away, Teresa's grandmother rediscovered an ingenuous freedom at the end. Velma no longer fought with herself or anyone else, something she had not experienced since the beginning of life. Losing the ability to walk was a discovery she shared with Kate. Teresa said they would hold hands and practice going up and down the halls of the nursing home. Velma was forgetting; Kate was learning, but mainly they were having a good time together.

After Velma was diagnosed with Alzheimer's disease, everyone in the family had braced for a hard end. When death came, it was like opening, then closing a window. Velma, having made amends for the problematic relationships of her past, drifted gently away. Years later, Teresa wrote about it:

> *In the last days, I took Kate and our newborn son, Adam, to see Grandma Velma. It was painful to see her so helpless. I remembered someone so different. I had always loved her so much. We sang to her, and we prayed with her. Kate climbed up into her bed and got right next to her. It was a moment I will not forget. My mother took the children to the car, and I told my grandmother I loved her. She whispered that she loved me, too. The next day, she could not speak. She died the day before Kate's third birthday.*

8

A Friend in the Late Stage:
Accepting and Honoring

DO THE REMEMBERING

INFANCY AND EARLY CHILDHOOD ARE the only times most of us experience unqualified love. When self-control, empathy, responsibility and other social skills are mastered, people hinge their positive feelings toward us on our consistent exercise of these capabilities, and rightly so. One of the ways in which late stage dementia echoes the first few years of life is in the need for the kind of patience and freely given love we bestow on a child. In a baby's fragility, we perceive the promise of years ahead. It is understandable to be with someone confined to a bed, unable to use his mind, and think to yourself not much is left. But what this person became through his work and relationships exists regardless of the fact he will end his life with advanced dementia. The extreme disabilities Alzheimer's disease imposes must be accepted. Continuing to love is a choice. Facing the disease without reassurance of enduring love and respect from others would add a preventable dimension to the anguish of the experience. When you are with a friend with dementia, deliberately see two people—the one afflicted by a devastating illness and the one who wore a white lab coat, raised children, played Brahms and Schubert, told stories, made the best cupcakes in the world, could argue a case, rewire a house, or design a garden. See the person you have always loved. A disease can change how the future will play out. It cannot change the past.

> *See the person you have always loved. A disease can change how the future will play out. It cannot change the past.*

HAVE REALISTIC EXPECTATIONS

A person in late AD may be capable of acknowledging you only in a very limited way—a faint smile, the lifting of a hand, an "ahhh," a glance in your direction—or not at all. Unlike Velma, most people near death are not speaking. Many are barely moving. This does not discount the importance of your visit. Bring along a book with pictures of something reminiscent of the past (horses, dogs, travel, cooking, sports) and flip through the pictures, talking quietly about them: "Ben, here's a terrier. I remember when you had a terrier named Scruffy. This Dalmatian has a lot of spots, doesn't he?" Or bring a photo album and tell your friend about the pictures: "Here we are at Easter, when your children were six and seven years old. Susan is wearing that brown velvet dress you made for her...."

Were you in high school together? Bring your yearbook. Did your friend enjoy poetry at one time? Longfellow and Wilde are rhythmic and beautiful to read, but any poem would be fine. The words won't matter; your presence will. Think back to show-and-tell in school and the interesting things you packed in a paper bag: "Aunt Juliet, here are the shells we found at the beach last week. Would you like to hold this one? Feel how smooth it is from the waves." Aunt Juliet will sense your care and positive intention, and that's what counts.

For another possibility, remember the longsuffering rabbit you once hid in your book bag and brought out, to the dismay of your third grade teacher and the delight of your peers? A well-mannered pet (unlike the average cat) might be the ticket to a splash of happiness if the caregiver has agreed in advance to a four-legged visitor.

Most of us have been stuck in awkward social situations when, out of the twenty-five thousand words we probably know, only about ten come to mind, and they aren't the right ten. Don't let the challenge of relating to a person bedridden by dementia leave you feeling tongue-tied. We strain to fill time, when we are uneasy, with ceaseless conversation. There's

> *By caring enough to be present, you will almost certainly lessen the pain of living with an immobile body and a shattered mind.*

no need for it with a friend in late stage AD. You can stop by with a book or a quiet project, sit by the bed, and say now and then, "I'm right beside you. I'll stay with you for a while." Play it by ear. It may be just as well to say nothing. Margaret, a caregiver whose father died of Alzheimer's disease, has this advice: "Go without an agenda. If you go into a setting, and you have no idea what to expect, but you're open to what unfolds, I think that's better." Whether you make an observable connection is not as important as the fact you will, by caring enough to be present, almost certainly lessen the pain of living with an immobile body and a shattered mind.

USE THE B•E•S•T WAY

Verbal communication stops before the ability to interpret nonverbal cues. One of the first connections an infant makes is between a soothing touch or tone of voice and relief from physical distress. A smile is associated with being held and cuddled, music with being rocked. People in late stage Alzheimer's sometimes find comfort in a soft blanket or stuffed toy that must bring back a sense of the security of early childhood. When words have lost meaning, nonverbal lines of communication will be left open. Remember the acronym "B-E-S-T" for ways you can continue to connect:

- **Body language.** Lean toward the person; keep your arms open, not crossed. Open your hands.

- **Expression.** Your facial expression can substitute for the warmth and affection you may not otherwise be able to convey. Smile if it feels natural. Even in the late stage, eye contact may be a way to connect. Try to let go of the expectation of a response. A caregiver, struggling with her mother's lack, ever, of any indication of awareness of her, asks in the anguish shared by many in this role, seldom acknowledged by the patient, "Does she understand me at all? Does she hear me? I want her to feel loved. I want to comfort her. I think that's the hardest thing." The woman continues to reach out to her mother, despite her discouragement, believing as a matter of faith that her mother is conscious on some deep level of her love.

- **Sounds.** Keep your voice quiet and modulated. Loudness can cause agitation and fear, since there is no comprehension of the words—the reaction is entirely to the tone. Talk about the past or your current feelings as though the person can understand, using the cadence of your voice to communicate. The meaning of the words is not relevant; the meaning *behind* them is: "Dad, I'm thinking of our first hunting trip. It was one my best times ever. You carried me on your shoulders, the mud was so deep getting to the duck blind." Calming music may be better than speech. Teresa, from the previous chapter, has a lovely voice and sang to her grandmother near the end.

- **Touch.** Touch can convey love and comfort almost more effectively than words at any stage of life. People—young, middle-aged, and old—differ, though, in their reactions to physical contact. If the person is pulling away or grimacing, he may not want to be touched. Take your cues from his nonverbal communication. Connection with a person in the late stage of dementia is based on simple things. Sitting in a sunny window, holding your friend's hand will be enough when he is no longer speaking. Think about yourself and what you most want when you're scared or lonely and in need of comfort—it's probably to be held. I remember sitting with my mother one night, when she was old and very sick. As a child, I would never have touched her hair for fear of dismantling the sculpted outcome of her twice-weekly trips to the beauty salon. But her hair hung like fibers of limp cotton then, and I held her close to me and ran my fingers through it. "Oh, honey, thank you," she said, "You have no idea...." She couldn't finish the sentence and silently shook her head, as if to emphasize my inability to comprehend what those few seconds had meant to her. Friends and loved ones in late stage dementia may not be able to show gratitude, even indirectly, for the comfort of your presence, but imagine that if they could still form the words or make the gestures to express to you their inmost needs for nurturing contact, they would.

ACCEPT "WHATEVER"

"Whatever," said with exasperation or resignation, is a popular way these days of letting a person know he has strayed into the realm of the unreasonable, but you'll go along with it for a while, realizing the futility of doing anything else. Let this idiom, rid of the smugness, guide you after your friend has lost his comprehension of the world around him and the capacity to control himself within it. The relationship will become one-sided, at least in the traditional sense of reciprocity.

The inmost rewards of selfless giving can't be measured by a tit-for-tat yardstick.[25] Kindness is a way of investing in your own heart; the dividends come from how you feel about yourself.

Cathy, a sixty-year-old with the look of a marathon runner, has found this to be true in her relationship with her lifelong friend, Janice, diagnosed in her fifties with younger-onset AD. "I thought I'd always have my best friend to bounce things off of, to listen to me and be with me. Janice is a friend I've known since I was a child. My grandmother and her grandmother looked after us when we were babies. When Janice started to have trouble with her memory, she seemed so quiet and distant. I didn't know what was going on. I thought I had done something to upset her, that she was mad at me. I've learned to accept the changes in her; it's very different. Although she's still in my life, I've lost her."

They have shared everything from grammar school and birthday parties to child rearing and divorce. "I remember going to spend the night at her house when we were little," Cathy recalls. "We would always have so much fun together, just doing silly things. Her mother was outgoing and fun loving. We played hide-and-go-seek with her—the three of us, on a school night!" As Janice sank deeper into dementia, Cathy realized those memories, drawn to the present in collaborative recollection, were the only place the two could be on equal footing. For a period in the disease, Janice's memory was sharper than Cathy's about their childhood.

Why does Cathy stay around? Because she knows Janice would do the same for her if the roles were reversed. The closest of our friendships deepen into love and commitment to see each other through the painful times along with the good, without emphasis on the evenness of exchange. Cathy is standing by Janice as her mind breaks down because her loyalty eclipses the difficulty. She's my friend," Cathy says simply. "I want to be there for her, but it's hard for me. I'm grieving, too. The loss on both sides is huge."

9

Help As Caregiving
Draws to a Close

ANTICIPATE AMBIVALENCE

JENNY, WHOSE MOTHER AWOKE from general anesthesia in a state of exacerbated dementia, said she passed by her parents' bedroom when her mother was near death. Her father was kneeling by the bed. "Please don't leave," he implored. "I'm not ready yet. Please don't leave. Not now." Jenny's father may have been the exception. People who have seen their loved ones suffer and have suffered themselves because of it seem to anticipate the end with bittersweet relief. The disease cannot strip a person of what she has done in the past, nor can it make a relationship, as lived over the continuity of many years, less precious. It can make death almost welcome, though.

You recall Sarah from chapter 7. Her mother was the beloved "wise owl" of the family. Sarah once said in such anguish and disbelief her voice was barely a whisper, "I wish she would die." No one could doubt Sarah's devotion to her mother. Her wish for her mother's death was at great emotional cost, but her faith made it seem like a release of the essential part of her mother from a long period of suffering to an afterlife freed from this burden.

A caregiver may vacillate between wishing her loved one would die and being sobered—perhaps frightened—by the finality of death and the lost chances, in whatever way, to connect. Allow the caregiver to talk without worrying about what you might think of her. Encourage it. "Let your friends say what they really feel," Sarah advises. "Listen with absolute acceptance. People don't want to admit that they would welcome death. Life is so precious. My mom loved life. But it's what you feel, and you can't help it. You hate the disease, and you hate what is happening." Giving a person the space to voice conflicting feelings helps to resolve them. Left unexpressed, troubling ambivalence can become one's own private, two-headed monster. When brought out in the open and accepted, such thoughts are less distressing. Consider these dialogues:

The Critical Friend

Friend: I started putting the rest of Joe's clothes in a box. The doctor told me it won't be long, maybe a few months. I hate to say I was relieved when I took his things out of the drawers. I don't know why I feel the way I do.

You: You're already clearing out his stuff? I can see why you'd be sad, not relieved.

Friend: I'm relieved he'll be out of this misery soon.

You: But do you want him to be *dead*?

Friend: He's losing everything. He can hardly swallow.

You: I know how bad it is. He isn't gone yet, though.

Friend: I guess I'm tired. I'm tired of paying so many bills from the nursing home. I'm tired of worrying about whether he's okay. I'm tired of

being called with problems. On the other ha
here feels like a gift. I wonder how it will be

You: Marriage is a challenge.

Friend: This isn't marriage.

You: He's the man you married for better, for worse
was always faithful to you. He was devoted! When Chuck left me, I
would have given anything for a husband like Joe.

The Compassionate Friend

Friend: I started putting some of Joe's clothes in a box. His doctor said
it won't be long. I was relieved when I took his things out of the
drawers. I don't understand what's going on with me.

You: You've both been through a true ordeal, especially in these last
couple of years.

Friend: Why would I feel this way? I should be more sad when my
husband is dying. I am sad to lose him, but he seemed to die a while
ago, really. I had a connection with him until this past spring. He
isn't responsive anymore. He hardly even looks at me or at anyone.

You: He has gotten totally debilitated. He's probably ready to go. Every-
body knows you love him, but he was devoted to you, too. When
Chuck left me, I would have given anything for a husband like Joe.
The two of you were so good together.

Friend: Maybe I don't feel sorry because I know he won't recover. Not
in this life. When we first got the diagnosis, I used to get up in the
middle of the night while he was asleep, sit in the kitchen with the
cat, and cry my eyes out.

You: You've grieved all along, and you've taken good care of him. He
would have done the same for you.

An emotionally laden mishmash of sleep deprivation, financial worries, never-ending chores, and the impending death of a loved one can make the most stable person testy. The positive steps that help with stress (so easy to suggest)—eating a healthy diet, getting more sleep, meditating, keeping up with medical care, exercise, social activity—can seem impossible when confronted by the constant needs of a family member with dementia. Caregiving at any point, but surely as it goes on year after year, can bring about a chronic case of frazzled nerves. Put on your social armor and let some things go, realizing your caregiving friend may be dealing with too much tension and worry to thank you properly for your help or even, at times, to stay well between the lines of common courtesy. Here's what can happen if you don't, and what can happen if you do:

The Supersensitive Friend

You: Celeste made extra dinner tonight, and I've brought it by for you. Where should I put it?

Friend: Just put it on the counter, please. I'm busy with Dad right now. I can't come out. Dad, wait. No, here. Not that way. Please swallow this. It's just a pill. Are you thirsty?

You: Did you say the counter?

Friend: Yes, the counter. Hold on; take a sip. No, don't grab or you'll spill it. Oh, no! Why did I use orange juice and not water? What a mess. Let me get a towel. Wait a minute, Dad.

You: The counter in the kitchen?

Friend: The long piece of Formica that's attached to the sink! Where else would you put food? On the piano?

You: Celeste worked hard on this dinner. She didn't have to. You might cut the sarcasm.

Friend: I didn't ask her to make dinner. I wish you and my father and everyone else would leave me alone.

You: Leave you alone? Okay. That won't be a problem. I'll pass that along.

The Compassionate Friend

Friend: Yes, the counter! The long skinny thing that connects the sink to the stove, where everybody in the world puts food!

You: [*Instant message to self: She doesn't usually act this way—she must be more stressed out than usual.*] Got it. I put the macaroni salad in the refrigerator and the rest on the long skinny thing.

Friend: Just a minute. I'll change the sheets later. Fred, I'm sorry I was cross. I haven't slept lately. I'm tired. I found out I can't get Dad in at Mockingbird Hill because they don't have an Alzheimer's unit anymore. On top of that, the dean called this morning to say Elizabeth has stopped going to classes. I can't reach her on her cell phone. I'm worried sick. I'd never want to upset you and Celeste. You've been so good to us.

You: Don't worry about Celeste and me. Can I help you find Elizabeth or sit with your father for a while, so you can call some of her friends?

TEND TO THE TEARS

We live in a stiff-upper-lip culture in which tears are supposed to be shed in private, and admittedly, restraint is often a prudent choice. Most of us have heard the mild admonition, "Now then, let's see a smile." We are embarrassed when our faces flush and crumple into a tragic mask of involuntary wrinkles. There's a quick clenching of teeth and often an effort to lighten the moment with humor. The idea of giving in to unbridled sobbing, a runny nose, swelling eyelids, and a dripping chin in the presence of anyone less intimate than a spouse (who has also seen us scream, drool in our sleep, and slog through several days of stomach flu) is discomfiting. Remedies to quickly banish the evidence of crying range from cold potato slices and witch hazel to chilled metal spoons for cupping over the eyes and ice masks.

Emotional tears, in contrast to the kind of tears we shed when peeling an onion, release anxiety and lead to relief. [26] Crying is good when you're with a close friend or loved one. If the caregiver needs to cry now and then and isn't mortified by it, just let him (or her) cry! Don't start clucking and hand over the tissues. Should you be compelled to dash to the guest room for a box of Puffs, you might say, "I'm not giving you tissues so you'll stop. Go ahead and cry. I may cry with you." You can't fix the problem, but you can be there, and you can gulp back any personal discomfort. Your turn will come.

ALLOW MADE-OVER MEMORIES

Death or imminent death prompts the need to reminisce, often looking back through rose-colored glasses. The threat of losing someone makes her most admirable qualities loom larger than life. We don't miss the peevish person who insisted on keeping the shelved books in alphabetical order; we miss the one who patiently glued our treasured glass ornaments back together after the cat knocked over the Christmas tree. Separating what you have loved in a person from what you have resented and focusing for a while on the good helps you come to terms with the hardest part of the loss.

Friend: Rudy was a wonderful husband to me. I'll miss him so much. Even with what I've had to deal with in the last five years, I could never have asked for a finer man to share my life. He was a saint—a true saint.

You: What are your best memories of Rudy? [*Instead of: What? Before he got sick, you couldn't stand the way he drank too much at parties. He never talked about anything but his model airplanes. He yelled at the dog, and he walked around the house in his underwear.*]

The caregiver may be trying to come to terms with a troubling past and the closing of any direct means of reconciliation. Even in strong families, where love and respect supersede the steady, inevitable hurts, repeated misunderstandings coalesce into oversensitivities, which can be piqued by ever-so-slight provocations—a certain look, a tone of voice, a flippant remark. Adult children sometimes harbor the hope that such issues can be brought into the open, acknowledged, and forgiven. Dementia takes away this chance. There will be no healing discussion that brings about a time, however brief, of shared sympathies. While AD eventually dismantles the long held contentions, the experience is more like losing everything in a house fire with no chance to rebuild or start afresh: Yes, you no longer have the furnace that never worked and sofa you wish you hadn't bought, but this is small compensation for the additional loss of irreplaceable albums and heirlooms you truly loved. A friend's willingness to listen can help put these regrets down and allow room for better memories to prevail.

Friend: I lost my mom way before she lost her mind. When she and my dad started having problems, she took it out on me. She was angry at everybody during those years.

You: You've been faithful to her through the dementia.

Friend: I know. It's better than it used to be growing up. Since she doesn't know who I am, she's more pleasant. I wish we could have had a good relationship. She got mad when I was thirteen and gave away my dog, Crackers. I never forgave her. I hated her. I think I still do, for that.

You: Because it still hurts. Maybe she couldn't take care of the dog anymore. [*Instead of: No wonder you hate her; what a horrible mother. Or: Get over it. You're fifty.*]

Friend: I took care of Crackers. I babysat to pay for his food. My mom never seemed very happy. When she was young, my grandpa dropped her dog off on a highway. It got hit and killed.

You: I guess she was doing the best she could.

VISIT TO VALIDATE

Many of us instinctively give this justification for not visiting a friend or relative deep in the woods of dementia: "I want to remember her as she was. I don't like seeing her the way she is now. It upsets me too much, and she won't know whether I've come by or not anyway." There are several good reasons to make the effort. First, the caregiver needs you to see what she is going through. Also, the person with dementia may behave oddly and won't remember your visit, but you will have given her the chance to feel briefly happy (like talking to a stranger in the seat next to you on a plane, who'll forget you after the flight). And, the memory of her dementia will not supplant the fond memories you have of her sending you cookies in college, helping you have a funeral for a dead turtle when you were eight, or nervously giving a toast at your wedding.

A salesman who had to quit his job and sell the dream home with a greenhouse and garden he and his wife built together to become instead "this stay at home person," tending to her as she slowly veered into the late stage of AD, said his children had no idea what he handled day in and day out. When his wife no longer recognized him, he found a lady friend, to their great consternation. Torn between his children, who rigidly disapproved, and the friend, who provided solace and companionship, he had made what he considered a life-affirming choice. His children, he believed, would have sympathized had they truly been aware of their mother's state, had they known what he faced every day in her care.

Trying to explain himself, he extended one hand, as though reaching for something. Gripping it with the other, he clasped both of his hands tightly in front of me. "If you hold out your hand," he began, and his eyes filled suddenly with tears, "you want her to hold it back. She's really alive. She smiles at you. She talks to you." He implored me with the gesture and the rush of emotion to see the importance of what he had lost. He wanted someone to care for him, and his wife no longer could. This man had fought in the frontline of a war, killing and witnessing his friends killed. He had learned not to talk about his emotional pain, for fear of recrimination. In caring for a spouse with Alzheimer's disease, he found himself facing the same isolation. "Don't talk," he said. "And don't tell. The friends you had don't know what to say to you. It's social niceties, no more. When you get tired of it, you say, 'To hell with these people! I don't need them.' But I do need them. I need them to see what I've had to deal with."

MAKE ROOM FOR GRIEF

Grief is like having a thing with sharp spines and a loud cry, a thing that doesn't sleep often, which comes to life in your heart. As time passes and it ages, the spines grow duller. It begins to wander off and for the

Grief demands indulgence and plenty of breathing room from one's friends.

most part moves on. For an interminable while, though, it is prickly, painful, and easily aroused. Grief demands indulgence and plenty of breathing room from one's friends.

Shortly after my husband's death, I spent a few weeks walking on a deserted winter beach, picking up broken shells. I considered the fragments of shells washed to shore in late fall storms, turning them over in my hands and carefully choosing only those which were broken in certain ways, ways that corresponded to my own brokenness. As the collection widened on the front porch of the cottage, my mother made a suggestion. "Keep these shells for a while," she said, as though having figured out how this should work, "but every day that you feel better, take one and throw it away, until they're gone." I could see why the idea seemed reasonable. The grief would go, one shell at a time. But needing, for an inexplicable reason, tangible symbols of this phase in my life, I kept the shells and laid them out like a cryptic diary on a long shelf in my bedroom. Now, a decade later, I look at them—this one, chosen because it had a hole in the middle and that one because the edges were jagged; this one because it had worn in the waves to a smooth nub and that one because it was blood red—and I see them as so many words, telling me how far I've come since those terrible days. The sea rolls in with comforting constancy. Grief ends.

Something in each of us, I think, impels the handling of grief and death by unique means, defying any preconceived notion of how these feelings should evolve. We do in grief whatever we can to restore balance, whether it is plunging into work, curling up in the closet every evening, or crying until our heads throb. People who are grieving need freedom to placate the spiny beast until it creeps away, so long as they refrain from hurting themselves or any other living creature. Give your friend's grief plenty of space and time to heal. The deeper the loss, the longer this takes. We are conditioned to put a good public face on most things, no matter how catastrophic. You can be sure that a person who faces a profound loss is suffering and will for a long while, whether the heartache is readily apparent or not.

PART FOUR

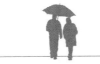

The All-Weather Friend

10

Willa and Bert's Story

What is dementia caregiving like when friends vanish? Here is one couple's story—compelling in love and devotion, disturbing as an example of the isolation that can too easily happen.

WHEN I FIRST SAW Willa and Bert together, they were strolling up a narrow street in a neighborhood where each lot has a well-kept clapboard house and a few shade trees. Leaves swirled in late autumn wind. Cars parked bumper to bumper made a tight chain along the sidewalk. From the back, the two had the look of accepted intimacy— the way they leaned toward each other, the way his hand guided her arm. They were talking, laughing occasionally.

They heard me approach and turned, and I was surprised by Bert. He was striking, with eyes like shallow ocean waters, vivid blue against the November sky. I had seen him before only in a conference room with the ceiling panels of fluorescent light that make most people appear wan and haggard, as though they may be recovering from the flu. He was there week after week for a couple of hours, his tall frame cramped in a folding metal chair, commiserating with other caregivers. Some days he seemed tired and quiet; others, he raked his hands through silver hair and talked about Willa. He had invited me over to meet her, and she gazed at me with expectation, smiling, uncertain of what to say.

She was a broad-shouldered woman then, with long red hair streaked in gray. Had she not been wearing eyeglasses pieced together with loops of cellophane tape, she could have walked straight from an Andrew Wyeth portrait of Helga. In her mid-sixties, Willa was the age a veteran of medicine's highest ranks might think of stepping away from the mandates and pressures to the calmer work of consulting. Considered during the Clinton administration for the post of Surgeon General, she should have had much to offer. But she couldn't remember anything about infectious disease or public health problems. She no longer knew her face in a mirror. Bert tended to her during those years as he would have a small child. "Willa is the love of my life," he still says.

> *Bert tended to her during those years as he would have a small child. "Willa is the love of my life," he still says.*

Back at the house, a width of nubby carpet, soiled and damp, ran over the porch, down the stairs, and across a strip of lawn to make a safe walkway on days slick with rain. Bert led Willa through the door and into the kitchen, where a box of disposable latex gloves, hand sanitizer, and rubbing alcohol seemed out of place alongside a rack of drying dishes. He hung his trench coat on the back of a chair, then unbuttoned Willa's jacket and slipped it off her shoulders. "Now, my dear, let's go back in here," he said and opened a thick Styrofoam partition placed against the door to the hallway. A handmade lock barred Willa from the stove, the chairs she could easily stumble over with the shuffling gait of dementia, and the door leading outside. She wandered into one of the two rooms where she lived during the middle phase of her dementia, restricted by gates and barriers.

Bert settled in a chair at the kitchen table, evidently relieved to have a visitor. Our conversation shifted quickly from books to Shakespeare, to nuclear energy, to his unabashed opinions about sex. "I miss having real conversations," he said. "Let me show you why." He stood up and walked to the gate. "Willa? Come here, Willa, and hand me your glass." He paused, waiting for a response. "The glass, honey, I'll put some milk in it."

Willa approached from her side and looked at him blankly. "My glass?"

"Yes, see that glass?" He could have reached the glass on a shelf beside a plate flecked with sandwich crumbs, but he spoke again to Willa. "Hand me your glass, dear."

Willa turned to a mirror on the opposite wall and looked at herself. "Well," she began patiently, "I've told you many times about it. What? How can I do everything? I can't, you know." Her tone was what it might have been less than a decade earlier when speaking to one of several hundred subordinates.

"The glass, Willa. The glass. Do you want some milk?"

Willa picked up an empty plastic tray. "I don't know. It looks like something spilled in there." She flipped the tray over and inspected the back.

Bert raised his voice. "The glass! Do you want some milk? Hand me the glass, Willa!"

Willa stepped forward and stared deliberately into his face for a few seconds. "I'm trying," she said quietly, as though addressing someone she considered slightly irrational.

"Just hand me the glass, honey. I can't reach it."

"I don't think it happened like that. That isn't what I told you."

Bert turned to me. "She'll never hand me the glass. She can't do it. She doesn't understand."

Willa picked up a child's alphabet puzzle and sang, "A-B-C-D-E-F-G-H-H-I-G-K-M-N." She set the puzzle down and gazed through a window. "What do you do with the man who said he had to go there, he says. Oh, that was very, very bad. That was very bad. Are you going to the end?" She raised her eyebrows in question. A framed photograph captioned *Queens University School of Medicine* hung on the wall beside her. One of a few women, Willa had stood in the second row, shoulders held back proudly, in the white coat of a newly minted physician. "Well, I am, too," she concluded, walking into the other room. "I don't know where I'm going to go, if I ever get here. That's the ditty, ditty, ditty, ditty, ditty, ditty, ditty."

Bert met Willa thirty years ago through his mother, a psychiatrist who hoped to lure her son from his solitary life as a West Coast journalist to the altogether different role of business manager for her medical practice on the opposite side of the country. Persuading him to make a three thousand mile relocation and career change, she realized, would require a more substantial enticement than maternal need. For this purpose, she put forward the strikingly beautiful and recently separated Willa, who asked only regarding Bert's suitability as a blind date, "Is he tall, and does he dance?"

Shortly after meeting the "gorgeous, brilliant, and interesting" Willa, the tall man who danced packed a van and headed for Florida, where a romance blossomed. A while later Willa changed positions, and the couple, inseparable by then, moved together to the District of Columbia.

"Almost every day was good," Bert said, reminiscing about that idyllic period. "We'd read to each other or just talk for hours. Saturday morning was the best. I'd go down and make us breakfast and bring it up to her, and we'd eat it in bed. And then we would make love." He talked about walking along the shores of the Potomac on weekend afternoons to watch Willa sailing a boat on the river. She was an avid sailor; he was not. Evenings, she went with him to a nightclub where he sang. "We were known as sweethearts," he said. "I'd always sing love songs to her."

Their lives went along tranquilly for many years, until Willa began to show signs of confusion and lack of initiative at work. Finally she was fired from her position as the director of a network of health services. In the stress of losing the career and lifestyle she loved, her dementia intensified. She was desperately aware, then, of her condition. Bert recalls having dinner with friends one evening. Willa abruptly left the table in frustration. She stood a few steps away and said, to no one in particular, "Please, please help me. Can someone please help me?"

As her mind faded, Bert simplified the love songs he sang to her, until at last they were only "ta-da-da" marching rhythms to keep time as they bounced a plastic beach ball back and forth in a simple game. While she could still play, Willa would bat at the ball with clumsy jerks, her body crouched forward in anticipation. She used to be a great table tennis player. When a psychological evaluation, required in response to her slipping job performance, first raised the question of Alzheimer's disease, Bert wrote an indignant rebuttal to her supervisor, concluding with the tongue-in-cheek claim that Willa could, furthermore, beat the psychologist or anyone else at Ping-Pong. He never mailed the letter.

EVEN AFTER WILLA HAD PASSED WELL INTO DEMENTIA, weekend mornings were a time of easy companionship, as they had always been before. One Saturday in winter, I watched the two of them resting on the bed after a walk. Willa lay with her arms stiffly at her sides and her chin tucked to her chest. A book review was being broadcast on television. Subtitles flashed across the bottom of the screen. She read sentence fragments and inserted them into her talk. "Gary Nash. Will we be able to get out of here? The unknown American. The unknown American? G, C … C-Span! C-Span. We hope we can grow with it," she said, laughing.

Even after Willa had passed well into dementia, weekend mornings were a time of easy companionship.

Bert's arm curved around the back of her pillow. Light from the window caught his eyes as he looked down gently at her face. "That's good, my dear."

When we were alone in the kitchen, he told me their sexual relations had ended four years earlier. "I had to work at it then because she was having some trouble. It was baffling to her, so I only tried again a time or two. She wasn't interested, and she didn't understand. There wasn't anything more to do. I lie next to her and hug her, but I wouldn't do anything sexual. She seems to enjoy being close to me. She's smiling and happy, but the relationship we had is gone. A diagnosis of Alzheimer's means you are going to lose the person you knew. She was my sweetheart, best friend, partner, entertainer, and helpmate." Other than affectionate touching, the only physical contact he has with Willa is in changing her incontinence pads, a task which was complicated by her resistant thrashing until her strength finally ebbed. "I'm glad she hasn't thought of spitting at me yet," he said ruefully. He takes these behaviors in stride, realizing they are a part of dementia but not of the Willa he loves. "Willa is so important to me," he added, "that to take care of her is to take care of myself."

A few months later, on a blustery March afternoon, he showed me the changes he had noted on a chart pinned to the kitchen wall. "Here, she could put on her own shoes," he said, turning back a page or two, "Now, she can't." He has used the chart from the beginning to keep track of her medications, daily schedule, and regressing abilities. Willa had been puttering in one of the back rooms with her hired caregiver, Becky, and we heard her cry out in distress. Bert glanced briefly in her direction and continued to read his notations. "You see, in the morning she's usually only wet, but the bed is flooded. "I've found that by using five absorbent pads in the Depends, urine doesn't get all the way up to the pillows, but I always have to do a load of laundry."

"Oh, stop it! STOP!" shouted Willa.

"Becky is probably trying to brush her hair," he said dismissively, as though outbursts of temper were an unremarkable part of daily life. After a few minutes Becky opened the kitchen gate. Willa was dressed in an overcoat and bright red gloves, with a scarf tied under her chin. "Hi, my dear!" he said. "You're going for a walk. How nice." He straightened her coat and turned to Becky. "I think this is a good idea. It's windy today." He took a tube of lip balm from his pocket and rubbed it on Willa's lips. They gave each other kisses, wiping their lips together in a ritual of affection. "That's the best way to put on ChapStick," he told me, in mock seriousness.

FOR AS LONG AS SHE COULD, Willa walked twice a day with either Bert or Becky, unable to go alone without getting lost. She ambled along, barely lifting her feet enough to clear the pavement. Bert had planed the soles of her tennis shoes to make tripping less likely. She kicked feebly at pine cones and rocks. She read license numbers from cars and words from street signs and seemed pleased with herself. She paused in front of a political sign in someone's yard one afternoon. "Stand...up... for...peace," she read slowly and turned to Bert with an eager smile. Encountering a stretch of rough road, she cried in the voice of a child, "Money, money...money, money, mon-eeee!" her voice stressing the end of the word in anxiety.

"That's mommy," he translated. "She's calling for her mother." He coached Willa constantly: *This way, my dear. Willa, let's turn here. Come with me. Good, that's good.*

Willa and Becky returned, and we sat around the kitchen table to share a favorite treat: butter pecan ice cream. Bert got paper bowls and plastic spoons out of the cupboard and took a tub of ice cream from the freezer. He opened the refrigerator door to show me labeled packages of cooked meat he had bought from a restaurant and saucepans of boiled peas and oatmeal—his method of squeezing the preparation of meals into the busy schedule of caregiving.

Becky scrutinized Willa from across the table. "Her hair has natural curl in it, but it's getting too long."

"I started cutting her hair when we were in St. Petersburg before we lived together," Bert said. "She was the only woman in the world whose hair I would cut. I had to be in love with her, and I had to have her naked." He laughed lightly at the memory. "I don't cut it anymore, but she got compliments when I did."

Impatient for her snack, Willa picked up the ice cream and took a bite straight out of the carton. "Very good, honey," he said with undaunted cheerfulness. "Now that's going to be your piece." He ladled around the tooth marks and flicked the scoopful into her bowl. Willa ignored it and took another bite from the carton. "Here, I'll give you this piece, too, my dear. Willa's very persistent when she wants something."

Becky offered her a spoon. "There, honey. You have a spoon for it. You don't have to eat it out of the carton. You have a spoon." Willa looked at her like she was speaking in Greek.

Becky cared for Willa several times a week during the middle phase of her dementia, so Bert could do the shopping and run errands. Otherwise he seldom went out. His efforts at holiday celebrations—a small Christmas tree stood in a window; a dozen dry Valentine roses drooped in a vase by the sink—were lost on Willa.

"Before she had this trouble, we were very much in love," he said once, as evening fell and darkness made the kitchen seem smaller. "I miss the way she was. She's very different, and I'm going through a grieving process. I know I've lost her; those times will never be back. But what hurts the most is for her to be brought so low that she has to be incontinent and live in this strange world. She used to be brilliant. I miss her companionship, and I suffer from the lack of that meaningful engagement in my life. I'm engaging with her, but it's very much in

> *"The love I've felt for her continues, but with a changed circumstance. I guess what I'm trying to say is, in a way, love does conquer all."*

the caregiving role. The love I've felt for her continues, I'm finding, but with a changed circumstance. I guess what I'm trying to say is, in a way, love does conquer all."

I DIDN'T SEE BERT AND WILLA again for more than two years. I was finishing the first draft of this book then, and I stopped by with a question for Bert. The same dingy carpet stretched from the sidewalk to the back door, but the barrier to the kitchen had been removed. Willa could no longer walk. She lay almost motionless in a reclining chair with her mouth gaping open and her eyes vacant. "Look, Willa," Bert said, shaking her foot and jostling her a little. "It's Mary. Can you look Willa? Look."

"Ma, ma, ma, ma, ma, ma," Willa mumbled, and the trace of a smile crossed her lips.

"That's it! There's a smile," said Bert and patted her shoulder. His voice had the same good-humored lilt, and his eyes had the same tenderness. He had pulled thick white socks over her hands, which were curled into tight fists. Without the socks, her fingernails, he said, would dig into her palms.

The whole scene was bleak: Willa wasting away in a room smelling of alcohol and soap, with packages of Depends stacked along the walls. The pages of Bert's chart were curled from use and filled with his notations about her. I wondered how she could be so thin and frail and be alive; how Bert could have carried on day after day, apparently without losing any of his affection for her. I imagined how different it would have been had friends been around regularly, bringing the outside world in and allowing him a break from the tedium.

Bert has lost touch with the friends he had before Willa's illness. Except for the Alzheimer's Association support group on Tuesdays and the company of paid caregivers, he has virtually no opportunity for significant social contact. "I tend to be in denial about how isolated I am, because I'm so self-sufficient," he said. "We're human beings, and we need to be in relationships with each other. You can't be great at tennis and keep playing against the backboard. You have to go out and hit back and forth with somebody. We do need each other. I understand that about myself."[27]

11

Seven Ways
to Stay Connected

EVERYDAY LIFE CAN BE A MARCH AGAINST TIME. We are only able to cram so many priorities into each ten- or twelve-hour window and feel the almost constant pressure of our obligations. Even in retirement, when deadlines are less compelling, the needs of a couple like Bert and Willa may look too huge and potentially troubling to motivate the effort of remaining in close contact. Excuses come readily to mind: "I want to help, but how will I make any real difference? Maybe I'll do something for them later." When embarrassment over a long delay in communication comes into play, that guilt-sparing *later* can unintentionally turn into *never*.

Don't be discouraged. Your company is a worthwhile gift for whatever amount of time you have. Think in this way: If a neighbor's house burned to the ground and you had an extra coat, you would offer it with no twinges of conscience over your inability to supply an entire wardrobe. Similarly, don't discount the value of twenty minutes to someone who lives with the demands and isolation of a serious medical condition. Do what you can, staying within the boundaries of your other commitments and emotional energy. You will be more able to help in the long run.

MOST OF THE SUGGESTIONS IN THIS CHAPTER are designed to provide support and companionship to the caregiver when the patient is either unable or unwilling to socialize. (The patient may, however, directly benefit from the first three.) Ways to stay close to a person in the middle and late stages of Alzheimer's are the focus of chapters 5 and 8, and getting along with a friend early on means responding compassionately to changing abilities, as discussed in chapter 2. After the disease escalates from the cluster of beginning symptoms to a virtual avalanche of problems in every arena, even your relationship with the caregiver, who is not experiencing the physical changes of illness, will become more challenging and complicated.

The caregiver's schedule must take priority. Our ideas of how to help, however well-intended, may not correspond to what is needed, so as a rule, don't forge ahead without asking first. I'm mindful of one day in the blur of days after I had stood in February snow and watched my husband's ashes lowered into the wet red clay of a cemetery plot. For a while I almost could not bear attending to the steady stream of people who stopped by, wanting—kindly—to express sympathy, although unable to grasp the intensity of my grief and loss. Some laughed and chatted with each other, perhaps in awkwardness. Some asked painful questions. One friend, a devotee of meditation, thought she could support me best with an unplanned visit during which we would sit together in silence. After more than an hour of her unwavering gaze in a living room congested with urns of wilting flowers, I wanted to tear out my hair. As the minutes dragged by and my attempts at small talk fell flat, my mother's past indoctrinations whirred like a private recording in the back of my mind: *Be polite, she means well. This cannot go on much longer.* She did mean well, and I felt bad about being ungrateful for such a generous outpouring of compassion.

In an extreme situation—and caregiving is definitely extreme—everyone involved is best served when communication is direct and free from social artifice and excessive niceness. Ask if having a specific help would be beneficial. Then work with the caregiver on the logistics, bearing in mind that caregivers are sometimes too inundated to be tactful. Says one woman in her early seventies, contending with both her husband's dementia and her own health problems, "I've become very impolite. I've had to forget about courtesies, like thank-you notes. I've had to let all of that go."

Rarely, a person deflects help as a matter of cultural conditioning or habit, as in: *Yes, but* the house is not clean; *yes, but* I couldn't leave anyone else with Sherman for two whole hours; *yes, but* company would upset my cat, and when Godzilla's upset, he shreds the drapes. In this case, forego any niggling swells of exasperation and respect your friend's right to call the shots.

Whether the ideas in this chapter are practical will depend on how the caregiver must adapt spontaneously to the patient's needs. As mentioned in chapter 3, the possibility of last-minute cancellation has to be part of the planning and extra time built in for delays. Caregivers almost universally report that everything takes longer than anticipated. Some suggestions may be impossible if the patient is going through a stint of aggressiveness or paranoia. Should the best laid plans fall flat, don't give up. It may take some fine-tuning. Here are seven ways to help:

1. WRITING THE RIGHT LETTER

Having a thoughtful letter tucked away in your bedside table to read in the middle of sleepless nights and times of discouragement is like having a flower that never shrivels into a brittle thread and a scattering of moldered petals. A carefully written letter cheers the heart over and over—each time it is read. We've realized the importance of writing sympathetic letters since ancient times. In April of 45 B.C., Cicero thanked a friend for a letter meant to comfort him following the untimely death of his daughter, responding, "… not only did you write what could assuage my grief, but in consoling me, you showed no small sorrow of your own."[28] Our forebears would be flabbergasted, perhaps dismayed, at the ease with which we now can dash off a few lines, hit "send," and be done with it. Opening an email message doesn't evoke quite the same pleasure as finding a squarish, hand-addressed envelope among the bills and ad flyers in the mailbox. When writing a letter of condolence, quicker is not necessarily better (although it's better than nothing). The efficiency of digital communication makes it more like speaking by phone. While email may be the best means of staying in touch with a distant friend, people long ago were forced by circumstance into hand-written letters, the more meaningful method of showing sympathy.

But what can be written to console a friend or relative who must stand by as a loved one goes through AD? Or to a person in the early stage who comprehends with real fear what the future holds? We fall back on the standard "you're in my thoughts and prayers," realizing correctly that this phrase achieved its status as a cliché by being safe and soothing enough. When you have the courage to write from your heart, the message will ultimately be right. Sincerity tends to be transparent and awkwardness gratefully overlooked. One of the sympathy letters I received came many months after my husband died, from a friend in England I hadn't seen since before I was married. She began a thoughtful letter, several pages long, with the lines, "How often I've tried to write you and torn up my efforts in frustration. I hardly know what to say." Two thousand years after Cicero thanked his friend, I shared his sentiment: It was comforting to know my friend had cared enough to try earnestly, realizing her effort to share my grief would make a difference to me.

Writing to a friend in the early stage. First, make sure the person with AD has been fully apprised of his condition and is comfortable with your knowledge of it. A caregiver, Betty, enlisted the support of her physician in using the phrase "memory loss" instead of "Alzheimer's disease" when speaking with her eighty-year-old husband. He had often confessed fear of the disease, and she felt he would be deeply and unnecessarily troubled by the terminology. They were both aghast when a meddlesome cousin deliberately revealed to him the unvarnished truth. Another caregiver said her husband felt distressed over the possibility his friends might learn of his AD. He chose to be seclusive when he could no longer conceal his difficulties. A person who is openly telling others would likely be cheered by a letter. A person who feels guarded about his privacy may not. Reading ability could have declined, but someone will probably be on hand to help. You might also enclose a photograph of the two of you together if you have one. Here's an example:

Dear Laura,

I saw your daughter, and she told me about your recent diagnosis. I'm writing to offer my love and support, which you've always had. [*Don't elaborate with assumptions about how she must feel unless you are in the early stage yourself and can speak from experience.*]

Your friendship is important to me, and I feel very sad to hear of your troubles. I still think about the good times we had in college, sharing that first apartment with your mom's old lawn furniture in the living room—and our weddings, both in the same month. I found the dress I wore in your wedding when I was cleaning out a closet. We've shared so many of the important events in our lives. [*Reaffirm your commitment to the relationship and relate a special long-term memory.*]

As prevalent as Alzheimer's disease is nowadays, anyone about our age could be in your shoes. When you want to talk, you know I'm only a phone call away. I can't, of course, completely understand what you are facing, but I can be a good listener. I'll be in touch soon to set a date when we can visit. I look forward to seeing you,

Laura; it will be good to catch up. [*If you make definite plans, phone just ahead of time to confirm. Your friend may have forgotten.*] Take care of yourself.

Love,

Constance

Although credit would be due for taking a stab at it, the following letter, roughly based on one I got while in the throes of deep sorrow, shows what not to write. Among other insensitivities, it underscores the difference between living with and without the restrictions imposed by a difficult circumstance.

Dear Eliza,

I heard about your condition at the Historical Vegetable Club meeting, where we've noticed your absence for many months and were grieved to learn the reason why. As I said to our fellow gardeners, you were brilliant over the years with bookkeeping for the annual cachepot sale and had such a winning way with difficult-to-graft cultivars. I know you must be depressed. Howard and I are so enjoying retirement. We've planned a bike trip to France next year, and I'm finally learning to play the Goldberg Variations.

Howard's beloved Aunt Edith Ann suffered from dementia and lived out her last years at Overlook Pond, which was lovely, but leaving her home was dreadful for her. I can appreciate how worried you are about the future. Of course all things happen for the best. I'm sure you'll find the strength to carry on. Please do not hesitate to call if there is anything I can do.

Yours,

Emma

Writing to a caregiver. Caregivers tending a loved one in the later stages of AD seldom see evidence that they are recognized or appreciated.

On rare occasions, the patient may have a lucid moment that restores, at least very briefly, a hint of the prior relationship. A daughter, whose mother was near death from AD, said her mother looked at her one day in the wise affectionate way she had throughout most of the younger woman's life and said, "I love you, honey." Then, just as quickly, she was gone again. A friend's written memories can return a person with dementia to his loved one, if not literally at least via the power of words and memory. When writing to the caregiver, try to restore a part of the person he has lost. Tell not only about the times you shared but who the person was deep down and what he meant to you. Here is an example of a letter from an old friend:

Dear Robert,

We missed you and Beth at the high school reunion last month. I know you are caring for her now, and the two of you can't get out much anymore. Many people asked about you. It's hard for us to believe she has dementia and is losing her memory, since we remember her so well.

At the reunion, they had posters of our yearbook pictures. There was a great shot of Beth with the cheerleading squad and another of her in French Club. I was always glad to be Beth's lab partner in science because I could count on getting a good grade. I accidentally spilled black ink from a fountain pen on her jacket in homeroom our senior year. Most girls would have been mad and told me to pay for it, but Beth turned up the sleeve so you couldn't see the spots. I didn't have much money then, and I've never forgotten her kindness.

My brother-in-law was diagnosed with Alzheimer's disease when he was seventy-three. Anne's sister took care of him at home for as long as she could, and she's not in good health herself. There are many people who have dementia now. That doesn't make life any easier for you. [*Remind the caregiver he's not alone. If you can, mention a similar circumstance within your own family circle—most of us have a family member with dementia.*] I wanted you to know I was thinking about you and Beth and thought you might like to talk sometime. My email address is goodfriend@abc.com or call me at 123–789–1234.

Best regards,

Worth

If you're a newer friend and did not know the caregiver's loved one before the illness, describe what you've gathered from pictures and stories.

Dear Sally,

I got your holiday letter and was sorry to read how much worse John's illness is since last year. The letter was upbeat, but I can see you are coping with tremendous responsibilities and loss.

I wish I had known John when he was younger. I could tell from the pictures around your house, when I visited, that your life with him has been exciting. I particularly like the photo of the two of you sailing on the Chesapeake. I hope thinking back to those times comforts you now. I saw John's etchings at Lakeside Gallery when I went there for an opening last spring. He loved the outdoors, didn't he? His talent and recognition as an artist are remarkable. [*When mentioning a talent or achievement, write in the present tense. A person's accomplishments remain his, whether he remembers them or not.*]

Although I haven't cared for someone with Alzheimer's disease, I took care of my sister for almost a year when she had cancer. She wasn't able to do much for herself. We could talk with each other, though. We were able to say goodbye. It has to be heartbreaking to lose that connection.

I admire your ability to laugh. I'm sure it wasn't really funny to have him bring you a ballpoint pen instead of a mop when you spilled a gallon of hummingbird nectar. We enjoy feeding and watching birds, too. It's wonderful you've thought of ways to help John stay engaged and active. [*Find strengths to compliment; many should be apparent. As mentioned previously, caregivers sometimes feel as though their efforts are not recognized.*]

Thank you for keeping me filled in. I care about you.

Fondly,

Hope

2. GIFTS AND GOOD DEEDS

Everyone has lobbed out the line "Let me know if I can help," realizing the chance of being asked for something specific would be slim. We might actually feel put upon if the recipient were to phone and say, "I got your note. Could you bring over dinner?" or "Can you come and sit with Sharon while I'm at my dental appointment next Tuesday at 1:45?" Our culture reinforces self-sufficiency, and in fairness, we are occasionally rebuffed in our attempts to help. All kinds of psychological stumbling blocks get in the way of accepting a hand with things—pride, cynicism, fear of imposing or indebtedness, embarrassment. When there is a clear need, perhaps the slight risk of feeling snubbed is a worthy one to take.

The first winter I spent as a widow, I had to drive three hundred miles in a blinding snowstorm to get home after a weekend further south. By the time I stopped for coffee, the headlights of my car were encased by a thick mantle of ice that spread across the hood and encroached on the windshield. In the shadows of evening, I could barely follow the road, much less make sense of the traffic crawling around me. I came out of the convenience store holding my coffee and was surprised to see a man squatting in front of the car with a metal scraper. He chipped ice away until two steady beams of light shone through the falling snow. Many years later, I remember the man's glance up at me and his quiet admonition, "Hard to drive like this, ma'am." His words and unsolicited help filled me in that moment with a restored sense that life is good. This chapter began with a suggestion to ask, instead of assuming what a person most needs, but there are exceptions. A woman stepping wearily from a motorized igloo was one of them, as would be some of the hardships of caregiving. Here are twelve things you could do with a measure of confidence that your kindness would be appreciated:

* *Do you have leftovers from dinner that will taste good reheated, like stroganoff or stew?* Drop a few servings by in a disposable container. *Have you grown fresh flowers or vegetables you could share?* Wash and prepare the vegetables, so they're "pot ready" or cook them yourself.

* *Is the caregiver's grass six inches high and sprouting seed heads?* Mow it when you can. Even a single time would help.

* *Is it the patient's birthday, or the caregiver's? Valentine's Day?* Take by a few brownies and some fresh ground coffee or gourmet bottled tea. Holidays can intensify a sense of loss and aloneness.

* *Is the walkway icy?* A fifty-pound bag of cracked corn purchased from the local livestock supply store may prevent an accident. Strewn on the ice, the sharp pieces will prevent slipping, and one bag can last for weeks. Birds will eat the corn as the ice melts.

* *Is the power out?* Offer to lay a fire; take over hot soup at night or coffee in the morning if you have a generator. Or just knock on the door and ask how things are.

* *Do you have articles of unstained, gently used clothing that are washable and easy to take on and off?* If you aren't wearing the clothes anymore and they fit the patient, drop over a few pieces ironed and folded. It will help when the laundry piles up.

* *Is the caregiver's car marooned in the driveway by a mechanical problem you can fix?* Go by with your tools and get the car up and running. A friend did this for me in a bone-chilling January gale after my brother's

death. I think I'll always remember with gratitude his frosty breath and very cold hands.

- *Do you worship at the same place?* Record the service and greetings from the members. The caregiver can watch when the patient is sleeping.

- *Do you have a book or DVD you particularly enjoyed?* Put it in a bag with a loaf of bread from the bakery or a box of microwave popcorn.

- *Did you and the patient ever share a vacation or past phase of life, like college, and do you have photographs?* Place them in an album and send it with a thinking-of-you card addressed to both the patient and caregiver.

- *Are you computer savvy?* Help the caregiver design a website she can use to keep her extended network of friends and family updated. At the time of this writing, a nonprofit organization, CaringBridge (www.CaringBridge.org), can help get such a website started.

- *Can you organize friends to help?* Look into starting a "Lotsa Helping Hands" community (www.lotsahelpinghands.com). Use the online tools to coordinate assistance from a group of friends. A link can also be found on the Alzheimer's Association website under the selection "We Can Help" on the homepage navigation bar.

3. MAKING A DO-IT-YOURSELF DVD

Commercially produced DVDs are available to entertain people with more advanced Alzheimer's disease, and they can provide a much needed break for the caregiver. "The weekends are the worst, because I can't get away," said Michael, a caregiver you'll meet in the next chapter. "Last Saturday I got a few videos from the Alzheimer's Association for my wife to watch, and it was great. I went downstairs to work on the computer. When I came back up, the first one had played through. It was snow on the screen, nothing else, and she was watching that. She watched one video after another for about three hours."

A few of the readymade programs are interactive. They simulate a conversation, with questions and brief pauses which encourage a response. Some include scenes and music from generations ago. Such materials can be purchased or borrowed from a library,* but if you have the equipment and software to produce a DVD yourself, make one for your loved one with Alzheimer's disease. It will not help him remember you, but this is a way to stay pleasantly connected while giving the caregiver a short break, possibly many times. Think of an adult version of *Mr. Rogers' Neighborhood*. You can watch an old episode on YouTube—note the way Mr. Rogers calmly, slowly engages his viewers. Personalize the story to your family and script it with the patient's memories, music, and dignity in mind:

* *Dramatize and videotape an activity he enjoyed as a child or young adult.* A few ideas are fishing or hunting, playing in the snow or at the beach, baking cookies with your daughter, using carpentry tools in a home workshop, gardening, tucking children in at night with a familiar bedtime story, feeding and playing with a dog, washing and waxing the car, hosting a child's birthday party, and taking care of a baby.

* *Get a thirty-minute recording of his favorite music.* Ask the caregiver for suggestions. The local Alzheimer's Association may have CDs to lend. Songs can also be downloaded from a service like iTunes.

* *Outline a script to accompany the activity or ad-lib with a few notes.* The following is a sample script for a birthday party:

Rebecca: (speaking in a slow and clear, but natural tone of voice): Hi, Patricia. I'm Rebecca. [*Instead of: "Hi, Grandmother, I'm Rebecca, your*

---

* See page 169, note 8 for information on Green-Field, the Alzheimer's Association's national library.

oldest daughter's middle daughter, the one between Nicole and Muffy." Giving details of the relationship to a person who can no longer remember you will be confusing.] We're having a birthday party today. Won't you join us? This is my family. Here's Dan, my husband. This is Suzie, my daughter. Suzie, wave at Miss Patricia. This is my son, Andy. Andy is six today. Welcome to our party. We're glad you could come.

Record five or ten minutes of table setting, blowing up balloons, icing the cake, and playing party games. Dub pleasant music over the children screaming, the balloons popping, and the dog barking.

Rebecca: Here's the birthday cake, chocolate cherry, Andy's favorite. Right, Andy? What's your favorite kind of cake, Patricia? [*Pause for about fifteen seconds.*] When I was a child, my favorite cake was caramel. Suzie, tell us your favorite kind of cake. Dan, what's your favorite cake? [*Stay on one subject; repeat it several times.*] Let's sing "Happy Birthday." Everyone sing along! Patricia, sing with us, too.... Andy, make a wish and blow out those candles before they melt wax on the cake. Yay! He did it. Go Andy!

Open four or five easy-to-identify, old fashioned presents, similar to those Patricia or her siblings may have received as a child.

Dan: Hey, Andy, you've got a yo-yo. That's pretty neat. I'll bet you had one when you were a girl, Patricia. I had one. Do you know how to use it, Andy? Let's show Patricia. And look, here's Mickey Mouse.

Andy: Who's Mickey Mouse?

Dan: You don't know who Mickey Mouse is? You poor child. Patricia probably remembers Mickey Mouse. Rebecca, did you watch Mickey Mouse cartoons when you were growing up?

Rebecca: Sure did. We always watched the Walt Disney Show.

To end, clear the table and wave goodbye. Close with a slide show of pictures or movie clips of birthday parties Patricia gave in the past for her children.

4. HOUR FOR HOUR

Caregivers can break away during the day if the patient, when at the stage of needing constant supervision, can be taken to a community care center for adults with dementia or a professional caregiver comes into the home to provide interim help. The hours are usually few and can evaporate in a frantic relay to the market, the pharmacy, the post office, the shopping mall, the bank, and the gas station. Caregivers, like everyone else, must run a legion of necessary errands. Crammed into one marathon session, it can seem like a quick sprint to the end of the world and back. Unlike others, caregivers cannot retreat wearily that evening to a good book, an uninterrupted movie, or an early bedtime. Caregiving continues around the clock and can be more demanding at night.

Identify a task you have in common with your friend, such as grocery shopping or buying a gift. Allow extra time, and while you are running the errand for yourself, do it for the caregiver, too. If you're going to be grocery shopping anyway, take your friend's list along. If you need to pick up a prescription, pick up her drugstore supplies as well. If you are taking the cat to the vet and know she has the same chore looming, make back-to-back appointments (unless a willing confinement in the car with two unacquainted cats would plunge you too deeply into martyrdom). Plan to finish around the time your friend drops her husband or parent at the center. Then you can meet at a coffee shop; transfer the groceries, the prescriptions, or the cat to her car; and spend the time together you have made possible by giving some of yours away. You may not often be able to add to your schedule, but keep the idea in mind and help when it's convenient.

5. TAKING ADVANTAGE OF TELEVISION

A television set can be transformed from a passive, rather dreary means of counteracting loneliness to a mood-lifting reprieve by the presence of a friend on the sofa and a bowl of popcorn on the coffee table. An enjoyable program enables the comfort of company contingent on no greater exertion as host or hostess than the click of a remote. Don't assume the person with AD would be upset by the animated screen, though some are. Patients may sleep at intervals during the day or entertain themselves with minimal attention for reasonable periods. Under the right circumstances, people with more advanced dementia may still enjoy watching familiar programs that remind them of the past, like *I Love Lucy* and *Bonanza*.

Maybe you like televised sporting events. Although high energy sports like football, which typically feature yelling crowds and announcers battling hysteria, could be agitating to a someone who lacks the ability to distinguish between physically present and broadcasted people, other sports—golf, tennis, and fishing among them—are relatively quiet. If you enjoy watching a suntanned person in expensive chinos whack a ball into the rough, as spectators clustered behind a rope frown in restrained silence, you might share this pleasure with a caregiver. Much of public television is free from booming voices, wild clapping, and shrieks of communal laughter. While *Antiques Road Show* may not be high on the list of riveting diversions, it is also not punctuated with the potentially disturbing noise of gunshots and sirens.

Could you and a caregiving friend find a peaceful show to watch together over a bowl of hot buttered popcorn? Indulgence can overcome the resistance to starting a new activity. You bring the popcorn; your friend can melt the butter.

6. VISITING BY PHONE

In a culture where people cannot seem to shop or drive without chatting on a sleek handheld computer connected to a vast communication grid, it is hard to believe anyone living outside a cattle ranch in North Dakota would feel isolated. Obviously, many do, despite the means we have of staying in contact, especially when they are grappling with a problem others find threatening. The more sophisticated and convenient the ways of communicating, the greater the despair of being alone. A caregiver unable to leave home or easily transport the patient sees cars pass and neighbors come and go. Isolation can be one of the most trying aspects of caregiving. "Going into a social situation now is not welcoming," says a caregiver whose husband depends on her for everything. "It doesn't make him feel good. He's uncomfortable. My world has shut down. We've quit everything. He won't let me leave him."

If you are unable to break the tedium with a visit in person, then a phone call is a perpetually convenient alternative. It's an available option when waiting in the slowest line of a supermarket or taking a walk. It's available if you are reclining at home on a La-Z-Boy, wearing striped pajamas.

Caregivers, like other full-time workers, may want to arrange it ahead of time, but a planned break to sit back and talk could provide a real opportunity to recharge. Here are a few suggestions:

- *Schedule your call if the caregiver needs advance notice.*

- *If you are concerned about being on the phone for too long, specify an ending time and respect the limits you've set by watching a clock.* The longest one person can listen nonstop to another talk, outside the context of a paid therapy session, is probably about thirty minutes. Most of us have a well-developed sense of give and take in conversation, and only the rare person prattles on incessantly without regard for cues indicating another's need for a break or equal time. The phone, however, eliminates the chance to give these signals, which for the most part are nonverbal. But remember that caregivers who have been alone for many, many, many hours with an adult unable to carry on a conversation are often longing to talk. You can give an invaluable gift by being willing to put your own problems and needs on hold and just listen for a while. As the time you have agreed upon draws to a close, interrupt gently: "It's 8:20, and I need to go by 8:30, like I mentioned. I'll look forward to talking again next Sunday. I'm glad we've found a way to connect."

- *Since you're not in therapy, consider pairing the call with a cup of coffee in the morning or a glass of port in the evening.* You'll feel more like you've met at a cozy spot in town, which matters when there's not much chance for the real thing.

- *Give the caregiver notice of a change in plans.* It's unfair to let any friend down after she has brewed a fresh cup of tea in anticipation of down time, much less one who already has a greater than an average share of reasons to feel annoyed.

7. SHARING MEALTIMES — THREE WAYS

Beyond the chicken casserole: a caregiver supper club. Almost every culture has a version of the chicken casserole in its broader definition as a popular staple that can be delivered in a disposable dish. There are times when arriving with comfort food on a friend's doorstep is the single best response to a demanding circumstance. To a caregiver trying to beat back loneliness, dinner away from home in the company of friends may be even more gratifying, but getting away for a couple of hours is often easier said than done for a person bogged down by responsibilities that fall outside common experience. It is considerably more difficult and expensive to find interim care for a cognitively challenged adult than to engage a sitter for a child.

This is how to bring about a supper club which accommodates the responsibilities of caregiving:

- *Find friends who want to help.* Try for a large enough group to allow for the inevitable conflicts.

- *Divide into pairs to stay with the patient for an evening.* On the designated date, two friends stay together with the patient, so the caregiver can go out with the rest of the group. Next time around, the pair who first kept the patient company joins the group, and another takes its place. The rotation continues until each person has spent an evening at the caregiver's home, and the caregiver has been able to take part in a number of social outings without the expense of hiring outside help.[29] As an alternative, supper club members could chip in on the cost of a professional caregiver.

- *Set a regular date, like the second Friday of each month, and choose whether to eat at different people's homes or a restaurant.* Cooking? Make enough so the caregiver can leave with dinner for the next night in disposable containers. Dining out? Settle in advance how the bill will be handled. Splitting a group bill accurately is often impossible without a flurry of fussy calculations at the end, and the less obtrusive method is to divide everything evenly. However, a caregiver or member attending singly should be spared the dilemma of paying a disproportionate share in a group otherwise composed of couples.

The caregiver must minimize the potential for problems by equipping himself with a fully charged cell phone and supplying activities to fill the time, such as photo albums or the type of DVD described earlier in this chapter. He should make sure the patient has eaten and visited the bathroom ahead of time. Behaviors that could be puzzling need to be explained. During one part of his dementia, a man who had kept western horses in his youth habitually cried "Montana!" when he wanted to be shown the way to the toilet. Being forewarned of such an idiosyncrasy, not easily interpreted by an outsider, would greatly lessen the risk of an unpleasant evening back at the house. If it works for everyone, the arrangement will give the caregiver a respite without an excessive expense and mitigate the stress an inexperienced person might feel tending alone to someone with advanced dementia.

This idea is feasible only if the patient can cope peacefully with a change in routine and is not likely to wander. If so, the caregiver would no doubt welcome relief on other occasions, as well. A friend who feels comfortable or is experienced in dementia caregiving could be a godsend at any time. Bear in mind that Alzheimer's patients in the mid-to-late stages, suffering from incontinence and sometimes prone to unpredictable behavior, may require specialized care and supervision a friend cannot adequately provide. Depending on the patient's needs and requirements, one of the ideas that follow may be more appropriate.

Take over takeout. Few people would be more grateful than a beleaguered caregiver for a takeout meal and the promise of a few hours of companionship. The options for prepared food are plentiful—supermarket hot bars, caterers, fast food chains. Almost every downtown street corner has a diner offering a convenient bite to eat that can be packaged as a to-go order. Here is how to take over takeout:

- *Schedule with the caregiver in advance.* Turn a blind eye to backsliding table manners and include the patient at dinner if he would like to join in. But don't hesitate to ask for what you prefer: "I've missed talking with you. Could we spend a couple of hours together, just the two of us? Does your husband go to bed or settle down by late evening and not require as much of your attention?" Understand, though, that as mentioned in chapter 5, patients with AD are sometimes anxious when the caregiver is out-of-sight, and finding a substantial window of time apart may be difficult.

- *Decide how to handle the expense.* For an occasional kindness, you might want to treat your friend. If you're planning to take food over regularly and need to share the cost, be upfront about it.

Plan a Baggie dinner. Have you ever thought about how many one-dish recipes could be made entirely of ingredients chopped or measured in advance and transported to a designated kitchen in multiple Baggies? A friend with a store-bought pizza crust and bottled sauce, and another with a few plastic bags of shredded mozzarella and toppings could visit a caregiver and quickly share an economical, no-fuss dinner. The same approach would apply to kabobs, omelets, salads, or any number of other creations. A casserole might work, as well as an antipasto or cheese and raw vegetable platter.[30] Add a carton of ice cream, maybe a glass of wine and the latest personal news, and you've restored connection, at least temporarily, between a homebound caregiver and the social scene.

THE OUTCOME OF A GOOD TIME for everyone, whether you are having a supper club or a Baggie dinner, depends to a degree on the caregiver's ability to set aside the stress, realizing that his friends' day-to-day concerns may not rival his. One caregiver, in unrelenting mental anguish over his wife's losses, reacted with anger at a neighbor for complaining about a trampled garden. His wife could no longer brush her teeth, much less grow flowers and vegetables. It was hard for him to live compatibly a stone's throw from people who were outwardly similar, when his problems seemed so much more serious in comparison. Another, with different needs, said she bakes chocolate chip cookies for the high school boy next door to entice him to stop by and tell her about his basketball games and girlfriends. Visiting with her young neighbor takes her mind off of her worries. Compartmentalizing stress is impossible for some caregivers. For others, a step back into an ordinary activity with friends is a welcome change.

12

A Different Dinner Party

Whatever's in these and those. And I think it wore me out then, too, that last time you heard me in stuff. I tried now, but then you'd never know. All our just getting their hope right. I tried to turn mine around. Goodness, goodness. A lot of the stickiness over there.

— ELAINE, *six years after her diagnosis with AD*

THE CAREGIVERS OF SPOUSES WITH DEMENTIA have a mutual regret: Dinner parties, supper clubs, and spontaneous evenings with friends cease; social life dwindles. The pleasure of being invited out as a couple is one of the many secondary losses with AD. Bert and Willa's isolation, described in chapter 10, is not surprising. "I understand it," says one caregiver. "My husband isn't easy to be around. I can hardly make out what he's saying. He can't speak clearly anymore." But I wondered if she was correct in assuming her friends would not want to spend time with her husband, an Ivy League-educated physician suffering from vascular dementia. How important is it that everyone who takes part in a get-together be able to participate in the usual manner? Or, stated another way, how hard is it for people to overcome their expectations of each other and let a different kind of occasion unfold? At best, a dinner party should be about helping everyone feel comfortable, whatever the contributions each guest brings to the table.

In the course of interviewing caregivers, I met an endearing woman with advanced AD, Elaine, and her husband, Michael, a community leader frequently called upon to speak at Alzheimer's Association educational functions. Michael is funny and engaging. Although Elaine's neurologist has confirmed that she is entering the final stage of the disease, she is mannerly and likes to be with people. She's unfailingly cheerful. I thought some of my friends would enjoy meeting her and Michael, so I planned a party to celebrate bringing the grill out of winter hibernation and invited them.

In the years following Elaine's diagnosis, she and Michael have found themselves closed out from their circle of friends. In Michael's experience, people don't choose to be around somebody with Alzheimer's disease. "They stay away, most of them," he says, talking about his friends and neighbors. "They'd rather go out with someone else. They don't want to be involved. And they certainly don't want to be friends. We can't reciprocate. How long can you go on in this one-way relationship? It's a problem nobody knows how to deal with. I'm living from one day to the next, but socially I'm not participating."

Because Elaine can no longer speak for herself, Michael suggested I tell the other guests about her condition when I phoned with the invitation. The across-the-board response was a disconcerted pause.[31] I could hear the sharply drawn breath, almost feel the mental rummage through the stash of plausible excuses. I hastily filled the silence. "Elaine's very pleasant," I reassured. "Her words don't exactly make sense, but just be natural and friendly around her. She'll understand that."

"Well," said my Aunt Nancy, "she doesn't sound so different from any of the rest of us." A few declined, but I was able to line up a full table.

As the date drew near, my optimism faltered. Now I realized why letting go of ingrained notions about entertaining is not such a snap. I balked at spending a tidy sum of cash to bring about an evening that might make friends, unaccustomed to being around a person with dementia, feel uncomfortable and in their awkwardness only add to Michael's sense of estrangement. The day of the party, as I vacuumed, stacked the clutter of mail and newspapers on the bar, and brushed dog hair from the sofa pillows, I felt stabs of regret. I arranged flowers for the table, chopped vegetables, rinsed the crystal and ironed napkins, worried I was on the brink of a hostess flop featuring long drawn-out gaps in conversation, made worse by audible throat clearing and silverware clinking.

I was surprised by my apprehension. How could I be writing a book on this subject and feel so hesitant? Why couldn't I trust my friends, including Elaine, to be happy for an evening out and capable of enjoying themselves without my fretting? By the time I caught my semi-dangerous cat and carried him squirming in protest to the basement for the evening, I was trying, despite this stern self-talk, to quash visions of us sitting around the table like strangers trapped together in a stalled elevator.

ELAINE WAS DIAGNOSED WITH AD in her late sixties. She depends on Michael to brush her teeth, bathe her, take her to the toilet, and dress her. He does her hair; he puts on her make-up. She speaks in gibberish. Michael is aware his wife's problems are the result of her disease, yet he struggles with the possibility of embarrassment over how she might behave in public. To his relief, she has not become contentious or paranoid. Throughout their forty-year marriage, Elaine has been good natured, weathering the tragic loss of a child and raising two others. Vestiges of her warmth and earlier beauty linger in a willing smile. She was the kind of person who would have rested a hand on your shoulder and made you feel fascinating, no matter how little you had to say. "Really?" her eyes still conveyed. "Tell me more about that!" She was the type you would look for if you went to a party by yourself and didn't know anyone there.

The first guest that night was my friend Steve. He bypassed the front door and went straight to the grill, lifting the cover and sorting through the tools. I knew that Steve, with a stepfather near death from dementia, would be sympathetic. Of equal value, he's an expert at barbecuing. I could give him a fork, a pair of tongs and whatever I wanted magically to reappear cooked on a platter, and no matter how the rest of the evening went, I would at least avoid the disaster of incinerated meat.

A FEW MINUTES BEFORE SEVEN, Michael and Elaine arrived. "Your directions were good," Michael said. "It was a beautiful drive." He handed me a bottle of wine in a gift bag.

"Well, I just don't know. The fellow with the chicken was here last night, but it's the doot-ta-doot-ta-doot-ta-doot!" said Elaine, dancing and swinging her arms around in rhythm. Her lipstick was on straight, and her clothes were ironed. She looked more pulled together than I did. No matter how hard I try to make throwing a party seem effortless, by the time the doorbell rings, I usually look like I've just staggered across the finish line of a marathon.

We went to the kitchen, and I poured Elaine a ginger ale. "Oh, thank you, the this and that and that and that!" she said. She held the glass carefully by the stem and took a sip. "My! That's the whole big wide one."

A fourth friend, Dennis, walked in while I was setting out appetizers. Dennis was formerly a world-ranked motorcycle racer with an entourage of fans who admired his intrepid style. Steve had been a professional athlete, besieged to the point of annoyance by flocks of adoring women in cities around the country. At about age fifty, if not before, most of us begin to lose the identities and abilities of youth. We find ourselves battling portliness, wrinkles, absentmindedness, hormone imbalances, weakening eyes, and arthritis. And, as we know, it only gets worse. Elaine had lost much more than her share.

Dennis shook Elaine's hand. "Aren't we ready to have everything go around backwards?" she asked enthusiastically.

"I guess you could say that," he replied with a smile.

Aunt Nancy and her daughter, Nancy Jo, whose mother-in-law is in the early stage of Alzheimer's disease, arrived last. Elaine clasped their hands, made eye contact and courteously said something about being flat on the weather, tapping into the social skills stored in the outer reaches of her brain, though conspicuously without the matching vocabulary. As Nancy Jo commented a few days after the party, Elaine was so efficiently going through the motions that if the evening had been watched as a silent film, she wouldn't have stood out in any particular way.

> *Elaine was so efficiently going through the motions that if the evening had been watched as a silent film, she wouldn't have stood out in any particular way.*

I overheard Elaine, as I put serving dishes on the bar. "I was going to be muddling through, and I don't know if it was a fellow and his wife, but one day the farmer came. Anyway, when they came on out, because we had just barely said to each other they're going to be hoping they can find her."

"Oh, is that right?" said Nancy Jo.

"I kept asking my own thoughts because like down there, they left this in that! You'd better think another time. I woke up for the laugh of it way back when they tried to elevate things around me here."

"Gosh, really?" Nancy Jo glanced at me skeptically, and I walked over.

"Is that snow on a white spot out there?" Elaine asked.

"Yes, it could be snow on the white spot," I replied to Elaine, repeating a few of her words. "Your mom looks pretty tonight, Nancy Jo. Is she feeling better?"

"Some. She goes back to her doctor next week."

"I didn't know that," Elaine exclaimed. "I wish I had, because we could have flown away if we had known. Oh, well. You can't always get away there."

"I wish I could fly away, too," I said to Elaine, then to Nancy Jo, "Would she want to make a trip to see my parents?"

"Maybe in the fall."

"I know they want to see her."

"Well, I'll be," Elaine said thoughtfully. "They didn't know when it couldn't happen."

"She wants to see them, too."

It wasn't so difficult. The conversation made sense to us. I think Elaine understood that she was a part of it. As discussed in chapter 6, much of communication occurs in facial expressions, eye contact, and tone of voice, and anyone can be included in those ways.

At dinner, I seated Michael at the head of the table with Elaine at his side, so he could help her without having to turn away from anyone else. She whistled a tune as she settled in her chair. He pointed out a few things on her plate. "See, that's fruit. I'll cut this for you. Here's your fork." Our talk drifted around between Nancy Jo's tennis season and the latest exploits of her teenage daughters, Dennis's recent family vacation in the Turks and Caicos, and Michael's upcoming trip to Scandinavia.

As Michael told us his traveling plans, I could sense his relief to be thinking only of himself for the first time in the years since Elaine's diagnosis. At a cost of more than two hundred dollars a day, he had arranged for her to stay in a respite care facility the weeks of his absence. His full recognition of her illness began when they were trying to pack for a family beach trip one summer. Elaine insisted on taking a wardrobe of winter clothes and nine purses. "You don't need this stuff," Michael had argued. "You don't need wool slacks at the beach." He relented and packed everything she had laid out, and Elaine spent the whole week folding and unfolding the clothes. Her family tried to entice her away from this ruminative behavior, which along with a tendency to dress improperly for the weather, is characteristic of mid-stage disease.

"Do you want to walk on the beach?" they would ask.

"I'm looking for my other purse," she'd reply. "Do you know where it is?"

When I brought in a tray of small cakes for dessert, Elaine reacted with a uniquely sensible remark. "Oh, that looks delicious," she said. "I'll have another one of those." She had sat quietly through dinner. She seems to know the difference between chitchat and earnest conversation, Michael says, and tends to fall silent when things take a more deliberate turn.

Afterward, we migrated to the living room, where my collie, Bells, lay at my feet, her eyes darting from person to person. We discussed children's plans following high school, and Dennis told us about his daughter's freshman year at college. Bells soon found a playmate in Elaine, who whistled at her. Delighted by this unambiguous invitation, she dashed across the room and jumped heavily into Elaine's lap.

"No! No!" Elaine shrieked, reasonably. "Not that way!"

The night wore on, and we found ourselves looking at our hands and the floor in front of our feet, without much left to say. I was thinking of the crusty plates stacked in the sink and the food to refrigerate. Elaine stood and looked around vaguely, as though trying to find her handbag or sweater. As Michael said goodbye and thanked everyone, I walked Elaine to the door. She paused and regarded her husband, lingering to talk more, with well-practiced indulgence. "There he goes again, there he goes again," she commented, then turned to me. "Have fun and tell her you're just going to bite your coffee." I reached out and held one of her hands for a second or two.

"I'm glad you came, Elaine."

"It wasn't yesterday when I found you can't try if your hair blows." She smiled and touched my arm.

In the end, I felt foolish for having worried about how my friends would respond to Elaine and whether it was right to invite her to a party where her difficulties would make her stand out. As Aunt Nancy had facetiously suggested, Elaine was not so dissimilar in some essential ways, despite her problems. If anything, she reminded us that as people with common frailties, we are inescapably vulnerable and in need of each other's care. With a little effort, we were able to change in a way that allowed Elaine, who could not change, to take part. And doing so did not lessen anyone's enjoyment. Rather than distracting us, her presence gave the evening meaning.

I've had many dinner parties over the years. This is the one which comes to mind as the best, and for the very reason that worried me in the beginning. We quickly got beyond any uneasiness and were able to focus on enjoying the food and each other. "I think that night meant something to everyone," Dennis said, much later.

> *With a little effort, we were able to change in a way that allowed Elaine, who could not change, to take part.*

There are certainly people with dementia who couldn't be integrated into such a gathering because they would find the noise and unfamiliar place disorienting. Some people who have passed beyond the stage of early memory loss require more support, like finger foods and lidded cups. Some, frustrated by the inability to communicate their needs effectively, become aggressive.

But often this is not the case. Shortly after having the party, I met a man with dementia who lives in a nursing home because he has no spouse, child, or close relative to help him with medications and meals. A professor of literature for more than thirty years, he can recite long poems in French and speak in captivating detail about Voltaire. He must temper his knowledge to accommodate the average person, and he is utterly miserable among the other residents, who for the most part have ceased comprehendible talk.

He described moving from an apartment, where he had lived alone for many years, to a highly regulated facility for people who need constant care. "Intellect is a disaster in a place like this," he said, sitting in a drab room with two single beds, no more than a few feet apart. His roommate is unable to speak a word. "Having an outstanding education is a burden. I'm very intelligent. Was. There are certain words I can't remember now. Certain words just won't come up, but to wind up in a place like this? Dear God! My life has truly ended. This is a nightmare. It's not anyone's fault, per se. It's the condition of my brain." The man could fit seamlessly into a dinner party like the one I gave and would enjoy the interaction. The other guests might not even be aware of his condition, although he cannot think clearly enough to care for himself.

BETSY PETERSON, A CAREGIVER TO HER HUSBAND for fourteen years, collected quotes from patients and caregivers. She provides these in her book, *Voices of Alzheimer's*. Consider this one, which might as easily have been shared by that French professor, Elaine, and countless others struggling with the losses of AD:

What do I want from you? What I need most is your continued love and support. It's not so much in your words, it's that you still care. That you recognize I'm alive. What I don't want is your sympathy. I still enjoy your company, conversations.... No matter how much I change, deep inside of me is still that love for you that will never fade away.[32]

I'll conclude with advice from a caregiver. Her father, a scientist who loved to grow flowers, died of Alzheimer's disease:

Be involved in whatever capacity you feel able and comfortable. Support the research in this field, hoping it will not happen to you or your children. And it is never too late. You can send notes or cards years later. I still like to hear stories about Daddy. I still like to see his daffodils growing in the garden. I think the worst thing you can do is nothing.

TIPS FOR A GATHERING

- Ask if the person with AD enjoys groups and does not become tired and restless. People who are beyond the early stage may respond better to a quiet occasion earlier in the day.

- For a guest with noticeable dementia, get permission to inform others in advance, so they know what to expect and how to help.

- If the caregiver thinks an entire evening might be too stressful, invite the couple to come just for the appetizers, the main course, or dessert. Give a generous window of time in which they can arrive.

- Reassure the caregiver that if an unanticipated problem arises, and she feels it would be best to leave, the evening will not be compromised for anyone—that you and the others will be glad for her to take part in whatever way she and her partner can. Should this happen, pack carry-out food in disposable containers.

- Try to plan so you can mingle and stay on hand to smooth out any mishaps, instead of being stranded in the kitchen laboring over a complicated entrée, or enlist another friend to help with cooking and serving in exchange for returning the favor at a later date.

No matter how it turns out, you've taken a chance and given your friends a gift of time and effort, a gift you would appreciate if you were in a similar place. Maybe, as well, you have helped others realize they can do the same.

BEYOND DEMENTIA—
A MAN AND TWO DOGS

The story that follows diverges from the main theme of Alzheimer's disease and friendship, but I feel it conveys a hopeful message, a reason for believing a loved one's dementia is not the final word, and is thus a fitting epilogue.

— M.C.

IN THE FIRST PAGES OF THIS BOOK, I described a personal loss different from dementia. The grief of it cut me off as surely as old age can, though I didn't have the furrows and sags, the thin voice, the stories told until they are like shoes with worn soles. I shared only the isolation many face at the close of life and the backward pull of better times. I remember looking at a woman in a train station and taking in the bones of her shoulders jutting from a hunched back, her spidery hands and faded eyes. I felt jealous. Every minute throbbed, and I could not imagine enduring the rest of my life.

I was in my early forties a decade ago. Bells, my dog, was almost two. I had named her well. She was joyful and loud. She tore the straps off of sandals, and she chewed cabinet corners. She learned to make a thrilling splash by tipping her water bowl with a quick turn of her paw. And, caught in the whims of recent puppyhood, she would not come when I called her. This annoyance was low on my list of priorities until late one night in November, when she ran away in the field behind my house. I stood in the dark wind, clutching my pajamas, screeching her name at the top of my lungs. Barely visible in the moonlight, she dashed by every minute or so, happily ignoring me. I finally tackled her. She yelped indignantly, and in our grim march back to the house, I mentally moved the situation to a different list—the one of problems I could actually solve. The next day, I enrolled her in obedience school. The only choice available was a class for the training of therapy dogs.

Seemingly, she then got what had been lacking. The collie is a working breed, so Bells needed a job. She sat studiously through the eight-week session, taking everything to heart in return for French bread with mayonnaise, the only treat she would eat after a nauseating ride in the car. The day of her certification, she performed twenty-one tasks flawlessly, including *come* and *stay*.

"Where would you like to visit with your collie?" a member of the committee in charge of placing therapy dogs asked, poising her pen over a form. "The pediatric cancer unit at the hospital, maybe? Children especially like collies."

"I want to work with old people," I said.

And so we did, at a stately brick building edged in mature English boxwoods, fittingly situated in an established city neighborhood. The residents were well-to-do, but many had lived through the Great Depression on farms, and many Depression era farms had collies. Occasionally someone would point a cane at me and squawk, "Come back here! What are you doing with my dog?!"

One man didn't say anything. He slumped in a wheelchair with his legs and arms folded into place like a made-up bed. His head lolled to one side, and a long string of drool swung from the corner of his mouth. I would walk up with Bells, and she'd sit quietly in front of him, as she was trained to do. "Oh, look, here's Bells!" his aide always exclaimed cheerfully, "Let's pet Bells." She'd lift the man's hand and place it on Bells' head, reminding him of his once great love for dogs. His hand would invariably drop off, as though it were a book placed too close to the edge of a table. She would pick his hand back up and hold it in place. Never once did his fingers move. He sat immobile, staring at the floor.

SOMEWHERE IN THOSE YEARS OF traveling the twelve miles to the center of town with Bells, I discovered she could ride in the front seat without getting sick, which made the drive around curving country roads much more pleasant for both of us. I bought her a special dog harness that threaded through the seat belt, so she would be safe. I'd strap her in, and she would sit beside me, her head about even in height with mine, glancing over now and then with the look of a person admitted at long last to her rightful station.

On our way to the nursing home one day, I rounded a bend in a stretch of road hemmed by a row of close trees and open fields. In the middle of the turn stood a golden retriever. Alarmed, I eased the car to the shoulder and got out, clapping my hands and calling. The dog trotted up willingly. When I opened the hatchback, she leaped into the cargo area of my car and settled in, evidently relieved someone had arrived on the scene to rescue her. She was wearing a collar with a phone number and the name "Honey." I drove off, thinking I'd drop her at a deli on a hill at the junction of the main route to town.

The plan didn't go smoothly at the store. Although the proprietor kindly agreed to take Honey and call her owner, Honey became suspicious when her free taxi failed to deliver her directly home. Her golden retriever smile withered, and her brow pulled into a worried frown. The store lady, seeing Honey's displeasure, spread her arms wide in what was meant to be a welcoming hug. Honey'd had enough. She jerked abruptly away, snapped her collar, and bolted toward the main road, where cars whizz along at fifty miles per hour. I grabbed a pair of bridle reins, which I had tossed on the front mat of my car a few days earlier, and ran after her, waving frantically at the traffic. Honey doubled back from the squealing of brakes, wheeled to face me and sat down in the parking lot, as though she needed a little private time to think things over. After a few anxious minutes, she apparently decided I was the least of several evils and walked resignedly to me. I looped the reins around her chest and forelegs and dragged her into the store.

We called Honey's owner, and I chatted with a couple of people at the checkout counter. Turning to leave, I stopped cold in my tracks and stared at my car. My knees grew weak, and my mouth went dry. The door to the passenger side was flung wide open to the busy road. I had neglected to shut it when I got the reins. I saw that I had also neglected to put Bells' harness on that day. Her white ruff lay flat and shining against her neck, without the crossings of black nylon. She looked at me calmly, having waited, sitting obediently, throughout the fifteen-minute ordeal.

"Good girl!" I said in relief. "Good girl, good girl!" I drove toward town, stunned at how close I had come to losing my own dog in this episode. I had recovered my composure by the time we reached the nursing home, but as I walked Bells around the block, I nonetheless felt shaken at having so narrowly escaped another catastrophe.

We entered glass doors leading to the main lobby, and I spotted the man, motionless in his wheelchair in the corridor. I led Bells beside him, expecting the silent downcast stare and paralytic body. Instead, he straightened and looked me keenly in the eye. I was startled to see the physician he had been, confident and quietly forceful. In a clear voice, he asked, "Are they both alright?"

WE NEVER REALLY KNOW WHEN perception changes or where people are within themselves. The worst tragedies are sometimes carefully masked; the seemingly unreachable in a person can be present in an instant. In this book, I encourage you, when you are with a friend who cannot remember your name or his own, to consciously see both the one in fierce struggle with a failing mind and the one for whom life was fresh and full of promise.

As a final word, let me suggest this: Look, as well, past the irreparable losses and be aware of a soul that can, I believe, continue on beyond what any of us are capable of knowing, disentangled from all that was enslaving and wrong. Whether you share this conviction or not, we are meant to pass through life in community with one another, helping and being helped when we are in need. Alzheimer's disease is a hard road to travel. Keep someone you love from traveling it alone.

MARY CAIL

NOTES

Preface

[1] See Ralph Waldo Emerson's essay, "Compensation," first published in 1841. The dementia Emerson suffered at the end of life, robbing him of his ability to think and speak, does nothing to diminish our admiration of his brilliance and enduring wisdom. Charles Eliot Norton, Emerson's close friend, wrote in a letter dated March 30, 1882 of having recently seen him, "his memory gone, his mind wavering, but his face pure and noble as ever, though with strange looks of perplexity wandering over it from time to time" (Charles Eliot Norton, *The Letters of Charles Eliot Norton with Biographical Comment by His Daughter Sara Norton and M. A. DeWolfe Howe,* Vol. 2, Boston & New York: Houghton Mifflin Company, 1913, p. 132).

About This Book

[2] Interchangeable for the purposes of this book, but not synonymous: Dementia is a symptom of overall mental decline which can have many causes, among them neurological disorders (for example AD, Parkinson's, and frontotemporal lobe dementia), multiple small strokes in the brain, infections, head injuries, and drug or alcohol abuse. A few causes of dementia are potentially reversible: depression, metabolic disorders (such as vitamin B12 deficiency), hydrocephalus (an accumulation of fluid in the brain), treatable tumors, hypothyroidism, and impairment from medication interactions and side effects. Alzheimer's disease is the most common form of dementia, accounting for 60 to 80 percent of all cases.

Alzheimer's 101

[3] See Alzheimer, p. 7,* for Jarvik and Greenson's translation of his 1907 synopsis of the presentation made to the 37th Conference of South-West German Psychiatrists in Tübingen, where he first described August Deter's case.

---

* The full citation of resources used for both text and notes can be found in Works Consulted, beginning on page 181.

The paper could not be translated literally from German to English. Jarvik and Greenson note that the word, "schneiden," interpreted in this passage as "to cut her open," could possibly mean "to ignore her." Their translation, however, is consistent with Alzheimer's medical chart and case notes on Deter.

[4] In the early 1900s, dementia patients did not have the support of medications to ease anxiety. We are also now aware of environmental modifications that can help calm people who struggle with their emotions.

[5] These diagnostic terms ("possible" and "probable") were proposed in 1984 by the Alzheimer's Association, then the Alzheimer's Disease and Related Disorders Association, and the National Institute of Neurological and Communicative Disorders and Stroke (NINCDS). A diagnosis of probable Alzheimer's disease is given when all other causes of a progressive, irreversible dementia have been ruled out. A diagnosis of possible Alzheimer's disease means that no other explanation for dementia can be found, but the symptoms are atypical of AD. The 1984 criteria were revised in 2011. The two classifications remain but were clarified and expanded to apply accurately to both clinical and research settings (McKhann et al., 2011, pp. 1–7 and McKhann et al., 1984, pp. 939–944).

Physicians use a battery of tests to arrive at a diagnosis. Steps taken generally include a complete neurological and physical examination, an evaluation of patient history and interviews with family members, tests of blood and spinal fluid, brain imaging studies, and neuropsychological testing. The process is rigorous and represents a physician's best judgment about the cause of symptoms.

An injectable imaging agent developed at the University of Pittsburgh, Pittsburgh Compound B or PIB, temporarily binds to plaques in the brain, making them visible in a Positron Emission Tomography (PET) scan (William E. Klunk et al., "Imaging Brain Amyloid in Alzheimer's Disease with Pittsburgh Compound-B," *Annals of Neurology* 55, no. 3, March 2004, pp. 306–319). In the spring of 2012, the U.S. Food and Drug Administration approved for clinical use a radioactive dye, Amyvid, which, like Compound-B, can reveal amyloid plaque buildup in the living brain by means of noninvasive brain scanning. While the drug may provide important information in ascertaining the cause of a patient's cognitive impairment and, possibly, in identifying AD in patients before the symptoms of dementia emerge, the FDA cautions that it should be used only as an adjunct to a full medical evaluation ("FDA Approves Imaging Drug Amyvid: Estimates Brain Amyloid Plaque Content in Patients with Cognitive Decline," FDA press release, April 10, 2012, http://1.usa.gov/HIrL3N).

Scientists are finding other ways to identify cellular pathology long before the onset of dementia. New diagnostic guidelines, issued by the Alzheimer's Association and the National Institute on Aging in 2011, specify a preclinical stage (mentioned on page 6) in which patients have no discernible memory loss and nonetheless show biomarkers, such as abnormal levels of tau and amyloid plaques in spinal fluid and shrinkage in selected regions of the brain, indicating that the disease is present. Earlier detection should result in more effective interventions and preventative strategies (Reisa A. Sperling et al., "Toward Defining the Preclinical Stages of Alzheimer's Disease: Recommendations from the National Institute on Aging—Alzheimer's Association Workgroups on Diagnostic Guidelines for Alzheimer's Disease," *Alzheimer's and Dementia* 7, no. 3, 2011, pp. 280–292).

[6] Alois Alzheimer's original medical file on Auguste Deter, in his own handwriting, was discovered in 1995 in the archives of the University of Frankfurt. In the 32-page document, Alzheimer transcribed in detail his interviews of Auguste and meticulously documented her behavior, varying emotional states, and physical condition, noting, for example, that she wore dentures. Cooperative during his examination of her, he reports she later screamed repeatedly, "I will not be cut. I do not cut myself." (Maurer et al., pp. 1547–48).

[7] Little information is available about Karl Deter. He and Auguste had one daughter. According to Konrad Maurer, coauthor with his wife, Ulrike, of *Alzheimer*, published in translation by Columbia University Press, Deter married the neighbor who aroused Auguste's suspicions (Strobel, p. 132).

[8] Condensing the pathology of AD into this broad brushstroke summary is like giving the following skimpy instructions for flying a jet: Get in the cockpit, talk to the control tower, push some buttons, and race loudly down a long strip of pavement until airborne. For books with a different aim and a more detailed explanation, try looking online at Green-Field Library's collection (www.alz.org/library/index.asp). Green-Field is a service of the Alzheimer's Association and is the largest library dedicated to AD and other forms of dementia in the country. Green-Field Library also offers the commercial respite care videos described in chapter 11. You may borrow materials through your local Alzheimer's Association chapter or a public library that participates in the interlibrary loan program.

[9] An important gene that heightens the risk of sporadic AD directs the functioning of apolipoprotein E or APOE, a protein that carries lipids in the bloodstream. The gene, discovered almost 20 years ago, has three alleles, or

forms: E2, E3, and E4. A copy of one allele is inherited from each parent—E2 is thought to lower the risk of the disease, E3 (the most common variant) is neutral, and E4 increases the risk. Getting a copy of E4 from each parent is the worst combination, but even such a worrisome pairing is not a reliable predictor. Auguste Deter's APOE genotype was E3/E3 (Manuel Graeber et al., "Histopathology and APOE Geneotype of the First Alzheimer Disease Patient, Auguste D." *Neurogenetics* 1, 1998, p. 226).

With advances in technology, scientists are finding additional genes tied to the common form of late-onset AD: In 2011 a large collaborative research effort conducted by the Alzheimer's Disease Genetics Consortium increased the number of genes implicated in sporadic AD ("Studies Find Additional New Genetic Risk Factors for Alzheimer's Disease," National Institutes of Health press release, April 4, 2011, www.nih.gov). Understanding the genetic factors which underpin the disease critically influences the design of clinical trials and the development of treatments and therapies.

A number of studies have linked sporadic AD to the same lifestyle factors that contribute to heart disease and diabetes: high blood pressure, elevated serum cholesterol levels, obesity, and lack of exercise. Even mild head injuries can heighten the risk (Victoria E. Johnson, William Stewart, and Douglas H. Smith, "Widespread Tau and Amyloid-Beta Pathology Many Years After a Single Traumatic Brain Injury in Humans," *Brain Pathology* 22, no. 2, March 2012, pp. 142–149). People with lower educational levels seem to be more vulnerable, perhaps because intellectual activity bolsters compensatory cognitive reserve (Catherine M. Roe et al., "Alzheimer Disease and Cognitive Reserve Variation of Educational Effect with Carbon 11-Labeled Pittsburgh Compound B Uptake," *Archives of Neurology* 65, no. 11, November 2008, pp. 1467–1471). Age-related declines in estrogen and testosterone have been implicated in some studies (Cynthia Gorney, "The Estrogen Dilemma," *The New York Times Sunday Magazine,* 18 April 2010, p. MM52 | Chu Leung-Wing et al., "Bioavailable Testosterone Predicts a Lower Risk of Alzheimer's Disease in Older Men," *Journal of Alzheimer's Disease* 21, no. 4, October 2010, pp. 1335–1345). For a summary of research on nongenetic (and potentially modifiable) risk factors, see Deborah E. Barnes and Kristine Yaffe, "The Projected Effect of Risk Factor Reduction on Alzheimer's Disease Prevalence" (*Lancet Neurology* 10, September 2011, pp. 819–28). Also see Christopher Patterson, "General Risk Factors for Dementia: A Systematic Review" (*Alzheimer's and Dementia* 3, no. 4, 2007, pp. 341–347).

The differences between healthy cognitive aging and early dementia, sometimes hard to articulate clearly, are outlined in a very readable paper by Rawan Tarawneh and David Holtzman ("The Clinical Problem of Symptomatic

Alzheimer Disease and Mild Cognitive Impairment," *Cold Spring Harbor Perspectives in Medicine* 5, no. 2, May 2012, http://1.usa.gov/168XK90).

[10] Current medications improve AD for about a year (sometimes less) in approximately half of the patients who take them. Pharmaceutical companies have focused much research on the development of drugs aimed at reducing, stabilizing, or preventing the formation of plaques in the brain. However, some scientists question whether plaques cause the symptoms of AD and suggest instead that dementia may be due to the harmful effects of free flowing, soluble amyloid-beta oligomers, which eventually aggregate into plaques; plaque formation may be the brain's attempt at sequestering these rogue compounds (Samuel Gandy et al., "Days to Criterion As an Indicator of Toxicity Associated with Human Alzheimer's Amyloid Beta Oligomers," *Annals of Neurology* 68, no. 2, August 2010, pp. 220–230 | Jim Schnabel, "Amyloid-Beta 'Oligomers' May Be Link to Alzheimer's Dementia," *The Dana Foundation,* 12 July 2010, www.dana.org | Cindy Sondag et al., "Beta Amyloid Oligomers and Fibrils Stimulate Differential Activation of Primary Microglia," *Journal of Neuroinflammation* 6, no. 1, January 2009, http://www.jneuroinflammation.com/content/6/1/1). The failure in clinical trials of drugs such as bapineuzumab ("bapi") seems to suggest, disappointingly, that diminishing the load of plaques in the brain does not improve cognition (Bill Berkrot, "Pfizer, J&J Scrap Alzheimer's Studies As Drug Fails," *Reuters,* 7 August 2012, www.reuters.com).

Scientists are forging ahead in the investigation of drugs formulated to inhibit amyloid-beta, despite the conflicting opinions on whether the target should be plaques or oligomers, and some encouraging results have been reported. Swedish researchers published the positive outcome of a three-year clinical trial to evaluate a vaccination for AD, called CAD106, which triggers an immune response against amyloid-beta, apparently without the potentially lethal side effect of meningoencephalitis observed in an earlier trial vaccination, AN1792. AN1792 is the drug Adelle (chapter 1) received before the trial was stopped for this reason (Bengt Winblad et al., "Safety, Tolerability, and Antibody Response of Active AB Immunotherapy with CAD106 in Patients with Alzheimer's Disease: Randomized, Double-Blind, Placebo-Controlled, First-in-Human Study," *The Lancet Neurology* 11, no. 7, July 2012, pp. 597–604).

For a discussion of the U.S. government's national plan to curb AD, which includes funding of research on a new insulin nasal spray treatment, listen to the PBS interview of Dr. Francis Collins, Director of NIH, and Eric Hall, CEO of Alzheimer's Foundation of America, "U.S. Launches National

Strategy to Combat Alzheimer's Disease" (PBS NewsHour, 15 May 2012, www.pbs.org/newshour/bb/health/jan-june12/alzheimers_05-15.html). Non-pharmaceutical treatment methods, such as deep brain stimulation, are under study also, so far with limited results (Susan Young, "Brain Pacemaker Tested on Alzheimer's Patients," *MIT Technology Review*, 7 December 2012, www.technologyreview.com/news/508461/brain-pacemaker-tested-on-alzheimers-patients/).

[11] Artist William Utermohlen's self-portraits, from the beginning of his career to the end, provide a striking visual portrayal of how Alzheimer's disease evolves (www.williamutermohlen.org). Utermohlen was diagnosed with Alzheimer's in 1995 and died nine years later. An article by Denise Grady and a slide show of the artist's self-portraits are available online ("Self-Portraits Chronicle a Descent into Alzheimer's Disease," *The New York Times*, 24 October 2006, http://nyti.ms/igxR4r). You can see within the anguished lines of Utermohlen's last portrait not only the scale of loss he had suffered by the close of his life but also, remarkably, the talent and emotion he was still capable of expressing then. The work validates the time honored saying *A picture is worth a thousand words* and, perhaps even more compellingly, gives voice to just four words Utermohlen could not otherwise say—*I am still here.*

[12] Age is the greatest risk factor for AD. One in eight people over age 65 has the disease, one in two people over age 85. As advances in health care increase the average life span, the prevalence of Alzheimer's disease is expected to rise. According to the Alzheimer's Association, at present a person develops diagnostic AD every 68 seconds. By the year 2050, the Association says the rate will increase to one new case every 33 seconds.

Chapter One

[13] For some patients, denial is a manifestation of frontal and parietal lobe dysfunction. The term *anosognosia* refers to a physical inability to perceive one's cognitive deficits and has been reported in up to 30 percent of patients with mild dementia (Sergio Starkstein et al., "Anosognosia Is a Significant Predictor of Apathy in Alzheimer's Disease," *Journal of Neuropsychiatry and Clinical Neurosciences* 22, no. 4, Fall 2010, www.neuro.psychiatryonline.org). See also Daniel C Mograbi et al, "Anosognosia in Alzheimer's Disease—the Petrified Self," *Consciousness and Cognition* 18, no. 4, December 2009, pp. 989–1003.

Chapter Two

[14] In the foreword of Cary Henderson's memoir, *Partial View: An Alzheimer's Journal* (Dallas: Southern Methodist University Press, 1998), his wife, Ruth, recalls seeing Henderson, a former history professor, struggling at the kitchen table to write as his language abilities failed. Henderson's book, transcribed from tape recordings and illustrated with artistic black and white photos by Nancy Andrews, gives a sad and touching firsthand view of life with mid-stage AD.

[15] See the October 9, 2009 entry, entitled "The Week," of Kris Bakowski's blog on coping with early onset Alzheimer's disease (www.creatingmemories. blogspot.com). Bakowski has been a nationally recognized advocate for people living with Alzheimer's disease for many years.

"Question to Clarify," p. 36, contains most of her blog, "Loneliness," published June 13, 2004. She concludes the entry with the poignant statement, "I see my friends going on about their lives, and I can't participate or I sense they don't want me to because I can't contribute. I don't blame them. They aren't being cruel. It's just life these days."

[16] Ralph Waldo Emerson's early symptoms are an example. Emerson was sitting under a tree with a friend one day, trying to escape the glaring midday sun. He noticed that his friend was not fully sheltered and remarked to him, "Isn't there too much heaven on you there?" Emerson began increasingly to use gestures and descriptions to substitute for words he could not recall, once identifying a dear friend, not by name but as "the mother of the wife of the young man—the tall man—the one who speaks so well" (*The Literary World: Choice Readings from the Best New Books, with Critical Reviews*, vol. 36, London: James Clarke & Company, 1887, p. 429).

[17] See Rabbi Wolpe's timeless, elegant book on grieving and loss (Wolpe, pp. 21–22). I felt comforted, even strengthened, by Wolpe's reflections, organized around themes of home, dreams, self, love, faith and life, during the difficult years following my husband's death.

Chapter Three

[18] See Ann Davidson's memoir chronicling a year of her husband's illness (Davidson, p. 36). Davidson provides a window into the experience of having one's life partner stricken by symptomatic AD while still fairly young. She tells of being on an airplane with her husband, on the way to an awards

ceremony where he was to be honored for his cutting edge research. He could not pronounce the word "coffee" to order it from a stewardess. Later, in his acceptance speech, he brought tears and laughter from the audience by describing himself, with a sense of humor ironically reminiscent of Ralph Waldo Emerson, as having a failing mind and an arthritic toe, but being in fine shape between the two.

[19] Henri Nouwen, a priest and former professor at Harvard, Yale, and Notre Dame, is one notable exception to this observation. Nouwen chose to leave his post at Harvard and spend the last part of his career and life taking care of a profoundly handicapped man named Adam. A prolific writer and philosopher, Nouwen enumerates Adam's gifts to him, not the reverse, and offers a compelling rebuttal of our societal tendency to base worthiness on mental ability and tangible achievement. He describes his friendship with Adam in his last book, completed just before his death, *Adam: God's Beloved* (New York: Orbis Books, 1997).

Chapter Four

[20] Many skilled nursing facilities provide age-appropriate activities, such as card games adapted to cognitive ability, scrapbooking, and easy jigsaw puzzles of scenic photographs. Although patients in the later stages of AD have abilities comparable to those of a small child, they have had, nonetheless, a lifetime of adult experiences and may perceive on some level the indignity in being seated at a community table, sharing crayons and coloring books. For an informative research study which compared levels of engagement in nursing home residents with dementia when presented childish toys, realistic and animated objects, or live babies and pets, see Jiska Cohen-Mansfield et al., "The Value of Social Attributes of Stimuli for Promoting Engagement in Persons with Dementia" (*The Journal of Nervous and Mental Disease* 198, no. 8, August 2010, pp. 586–592).

Chapter Five

[21] A person in mid-stage dementia needs longer than we typically allow to process verbal messages. You may need to wait for 15 seconds or more to give sufficient time for a response. Keep your statements and questions simple and concrete.

[22] Alzheimer's patients have varying speech and language difficulties at different points in the disease. All patients do not eventually speak in fluent,

monological jargon—described here as "word salad." This symptom closely resembles a form of aphasia (loss of language abilities without loss of intellect) associated with damage to the left temporal lobe: Sentences are produced with appropriate intonation, but they make little or no sense (see p. 151). Early in the disease, a majority of patients experience naming deficits, in which speech is essentially normal but limited by an impairment in word-finding, hence the reliance on word substitutions and descriptive phrases ("the things I wear on my feet" for "shoes"). Later in the disease, speech may become perseverative or echolalic. In the end, it ceases altogether. For a discussion comparing the case studies of Carl Wernike, a German neurologist who linked language deficiencies to specific lesions in the brain, to the case studies of Alois Alzheimer, see P. J. Matthews et al., "Wenicke and Alzheimer on the Language Disturbances of Dementia and Aphasia" (*Brain and Language* 46, no. 3, April 1994, pp. 439–462).

Chapter Seven

[23] Alzheimer's disease is the sixth leading cause of death in the United States. If the patient survives to the very end, she will have difficulty swallowing and can aspirate foreign material into the lungs, leading to pneumonia. Death frequently happens at an earlier point in the disease from complications of dementia. Bedsores, which you'll recall contributed to Auguste Deter's death, are caused by immobility; urinary tract infection is a risk with incontinence; the inability to coordinate the motions of walking or the skills needed to drive safely can result in serious injury. Without the capacity to speak coherently, a patient cannot report early symptoms of a secondary illness or actively participate in her care. Lacking comprehension of both time and risk, she cannot manage medications responsibly or stay out of dangerous situations.

[24] For current research on the effects of certain types of general anesthesia on Alzheimer's disease, see in particular the work of Dr. Zhongcong Xie, Director of the Geriatric Anesthesia Research Unit, Harvard Medical School. Xie is one of ten authors of a study comparing the safety for AD patients of two common anesthetics (Z. Yiying et al., "Anesthetics Isoflurane and Desflurane Differently Affect Mitochondrial Function, Learning, and Memory," *Annals of Neurology* 71, no. 5, May 2012, pp. 687–698). To access a link to the abstract of this article, which may be helpful if you would like to discuss the concern with a physician, use www.onlinelibrary.wiley.com; enter the article title into the advanced search box.

Chapter Eight

[25] Novelist Henry James, whose writing can seem at times deliberately complex, gave his nephew this famous advice: "Three things in human life are important. The first is to be kind. The second is to be kind. The third is to be kind." A century later, a number of scientific studies validate the claim. Researchers have found that counting and recording one's kindnesses for a week significantly increases feelings of happiness (Keiko Otake et al., "Happy People Become Happier Through Kindness: A Counting Kindness Intervention," *Journal of Happiness Studies* 7, no. 3, September 2006, pp. 361–375). Similarly, Dr. Stephen Post, of Case Western Reserve University, correlated compassion with both longevity and a sense of well-being, provided that helping behavior is kept within reasonable limits. The emerging science of love and giving is summarized in his book, *Why Good Things Happen to Good People: How to Live a Longer, Healthier, Happier Life by the Simple Act of Giving,* coauthored by Jill Neimark and Otis Moss, Jr. (New York: Broadway Books, 2008).

Chapter Nine

[26] Lacrimal glands of the eyes produce three types of tears—basal tears, which keep the eyes hydrated; reflex tears, which flush out irritants; and emotional tears. Emotional tears have a different composition than other tears. They contain enkephalin, a pain relieving endorphin, and prolactin, a hormone which affects immune response and reproductive processes. People feel better after crying because tears wash away chemicals produced in excess during times of stress. See Dr. William Frey and Murial Langseth's *Crying: The Mystery of Tears* (New York: HarperCollins Publishers, 1985) and also an interesting article by Pam Belluck, "In Women's Tears, a Chemical That Says, 'Not Tonight, Dear'" (*The New York Times,* 7 January 2011, p. A5).

Science aside, Charles Dickens may have said it best in *Great Expectations,* as the main character struggles with moving away from his childhood home, his harsh experience there notwithstanding: "Heaven knows we need never be ashamed of our tears, for they are the rain upon the blinding dust of earth overlying our hard hearts" (*Great Expectations: A Norton Critical Edition,* ed. Edgar Rosenberg, New York: W.W. Norton & Company, 1999, p. 116).

Chapter Ten

[27] Willa died on April 13, 2011. Her final diagnosis was small stroke or vascular dementia, although for ten years she exemplified the classic behaviors and stage-related changes of AD.

Chapter Eleven

[28] Cicero's letter begins, "Yes, Servius, I could, indeed, have wished, as you say, that you had been by my side in my most grievous affliction. How much you could have helped, had you been with me ... I can easily understand from the feeling of greater tranquility which your letter gave me" (Cicero, *The Letters to His Friends,* Vol. 1, translated by W. Glynn Williams, Cambridge, Mass.: Harvard University Press, 1958, p. 227).

[29] A supper club may also be helpful to patient-and-caregiver couples in retirement communities. It can seem wrong to leave a spouse staying in a separate unit, which provides more intensive care, alone at mealtimes. Continually missing meals with the larger group may bring on a sense of loneliness even in a setting with built-in opportunities for socializing.

[30] For Baggie dinner ideas, look at some of the limited ingredient cookbooks. Gooseberry Patch's *5 Ingredients or Less Cookbook* (www.gooseberrypatch.com), has many recipes friends could assemble with ease. *Cooking Light* and *Better Homes and Gardens* have published five-ingredient cookbooks, too.

Chapter Twelve

[31] Hesitation on the part of my prospective guests was, of course, due to social awkwardness and uncertainty about how the evening might play out and not to the fear of somehow contracting the disease. Along these lines, however, media reports of late have summarized research showing that certain of the brain abnormalities of AD can be initiated by injecting brain extracts containing small amounts of amyloid-beta directly into the brains of genetically engineered mice and that the tangling of tau protein can spread sequentially from neuron to neuron (Jamie Talen, "Two Labs, Same Conclusion," *Neurology Today* 12, no. 6, March 2012, pp. 1, 22–24 | Liu L. Drouet et al., "Trans-synaptic Spread of Tau Pathology in Vivo," *PLOS One* 7, no. 2, 2012, http://bit.ly/zJfeki | Lary C. Walker and Harry

LeVine III, "Corruption and Spread of Pathogenic Protein Seeding in Neurodegenerative Disorders," *Journal of Biological Chemistry* 287, September 2012, pp. 33109–33115).

These and similar studies have prompted a flurry of media reports captioned "Is Alzheimer's Disease Contagious?" and raised the threat of AD's similarity to mad cow disease, linked, we know, to invasive, treatment-defying prions, which are contractible by eating contaminated meat. The problem created by the use of such words in the press as "prion" and "contagious," at least for the headline skimmers among us, is our tendency to find too quickly within them the justification for a leap of logic onto the notion that we can, by avoiding everyday exposures, limit our own vulnerability to the disease. Even without benefit of corroborating science, we must come to the commonsense conclusion that if Alzheimer's disease were transmittable by any form of normal human contact, family caregivers engaged in the intimate care of their loved ones would fall victim to it as a result, and they don't.

It seems the main layperson takeaway from these studies should be the hope they will generate therapeutic methods aimed at a different, perhaps more effective point of intervention. That said, I recommend two resources for those who wish to learn more: a refreshingly accessible article by John Hardy and Tamas Revesz ("The Spread of Neurodegenerative Diseases," *New England Journal of Medicine* 366, no. 22, 31 May 2012, pp. 2126–2128) and the *Neurology Today* podcast, "Does Alzheimer's Disease Spread in the Brain?" featuring an interview with Bradley Hyman, of Harvard Medical School, and Karen Duff, of Columbia University, who briefly explain how research developments in this area may lead to new approaches to treatment (Jamie Talen, February 29, 2012, http://bit.ly/rCBryX).

[32] See Betsy Peterson's *Voices of Alzheimer's: Courage, Hope, and Love in the Face of Dementia,* page 46. Peterson's husband was diagnosed with probable Alzheimer's at the age of 72, shortly before their tenth wedding anniversary. In the book's introduction, Peterson tells of her own diagnosis of breast cancer after moving her husband to an assisted living facility. He died several weeks after her final chemotherapy treatment. She notes the contrast between the practical outpouring of support her friends offered during her treatment and their considerably more subdued response to her husband's very different illness.

Reading her book is almost like taking part vicariously in an Alzheimer's support group. Quotations, seemingly chosen for inclusion in the book because they are widely representative, are organized around headings of friendship, loneliness, finances, dignity, and other relevant topics commonly discussed in these groups.

FURTHER READING

The following is a brief list of reading materials you may find particularly helpful in understanding the experience and losses of Alzheimer's disease:

Brackey, Jolene. *Creating Moments of Joy: A Journal for Caregivers*. West Lafayette, Ind.: Purdue University Press, 2008.

DeBaggio, Thomas. *When It Gets Dark: An Enlightened Reflection on Life with Alzheimer's*. New York: The Free Press, 2007.

Doraiswamy, P. Murali, Lisa P Gwyther, and Tina Adler. *The Alzheimer's Action Plan: What You Need to Know—and What You Can Do—About Memory Problems, from Prevention to Early Intervention and Care*. New York: St. Martin's Griffin, 2009.*

Franzen, Jonathan. "My Father's Brain: What Alzheimer's Takes Away." *The New Yorker* (September 10, 2001): 81–91. (Note: An older article but well worth locating—generally available in *The New Yorker* archives.)

Genova, Lisa. *Still Alice*. New York: Gallery Books, 2009.

Grady, Denise. "When Illness Makes a Spouse a Stranger." *The New York Times*. 5 May 2012, www.nytimes.com. (Note: This article is about a man who has frontotemporal lobe dementia, not AD, and his wife's care of him. It beautifully, movingly captures the loss, fear, frustration and transformations of love caregivers experience, whatever the cause of dementia.)*

Hadas, Rachel. *Strange Relation: A Memoir of Marriage, Dementia, and Poetry*. Philadelphia: Paul Dry Books, 2011.

Henderson, Carey. *Partial View: An Alzheimer's Journal*. Dallas: Southern Methodist University Press, 1998.

Kleinman, Arthur. "Forum: On Caregiving." *Harvard Magazine* 112, no. 6 (July–August 2010): 25–29.

* *Also listed in Works Consulted.*

Marcell, Jacqueline. *Elder Rage, or Take My Father ... Please!: How to Survive Caring for Elderly Parents.* Irvine, Calif.: Impressive Press, 2001.

Miller, Sue. *The Story of My Father: A Memoir.* New York: Random House, 2004.

Mitchell, Marilyn. *Dancing on Quicksand: A Gift of Friendship in the Age of Alzheimer's.* Boulder: Colo.: Johnson Books, 2002.

Petersen, Barry. *Jan's Story: Love Lost to the Long Goodbye of Alzheimer's.* North Fayette, Pa.: Behler Publications, 2010.

Peterson, Betsy. *Voices of Alzheimer's: Courage, Hope, and Love in the Face of Dementia.* Philadelphia: DaCapo Life Long, 2004.*

Shenk, David. *The Forgetting: Alzheimer's: Portrait of an Epidemic.* New York: Anchor Books, 2003.

Shriver, Maria. *What's Happening to Grandpa?* New York: Little, Brown Books for Young Readers, 2004.

Simpson, Robert and Anne Simpson. *Through the Wilderness of Alzheimer's: A Guide in Two Voices.* Minneapolis: Augsburg Fortress, 1999.

Sittser, Gerald L. *A Grace Disguised: How the Soul Grows Through Loss.* Grand Rapids, Mich.: Zondervan Publishing House, 1995. (Note: Like David Wolpe's *Making Loss Matter,* listed below, this book is not about Alzheimer's disease. It is Sittser's honest, searing account of his grief following a tragic accident that claimed the lives of three family members. Sittser does not evade the hard questions we ask, when confronted by terrible, seemingly random loss, nor does he offer easy answers. His willingness to face these enigmas with intelligent thought is transformative and ultimately hopeful. Alzheimer's disease is a different kind of loss. However, the questions—*Why me? Where is God? How will life go on?*—and the upending of life, Sittser says, happen whether a loss is sudden, like a flood caused by a broken dam, or gradual, like the same flood brought on by ceaseless rain.)

Taylor, Richard. *Alzheimer's from the Inside Out.* Baltimore: Health Professions Press, 2007.

Wolpe, David. *Making Loss Matter: Creating Meaning in Difficult Times.* New York: Riverhead Books, 1999.*

ACKNOWLEDGEMENTS

I HAVE AN INCOMPLETE LIST of people to thank, without whom this book would not have been possible. My father, Jack P. McDaniel, M.D., read drafts over and over again, marking the sections he particularly liked. He beamed and told me unconditionally how wonderful the book was, even during my rough starts, which were hardly deserving of praise. Equally I thank my mother, Janice McDaniel, for her indispensable support and lifelong friendship.

I gratefully acknowledge, as well, the following people:

Willa M. Brown, M.D., is "Willa" of chapter 10, one of only a few people accurately named in the book. Willa spent her life as a public health administrator helping disenfranchised people secure medical care. Bert Brown, her husband and caregiver, let me sit in their home for days; he held back nothing in his descriptions of Willa, their marriage, her downturn into dementia, and his own sense of loss. Many people, whose names I changed for the sake of privacy, shared with comparable generosity in the writing of this book. Their stories fill the pages and inform the strategies and suggestions. Bert, however, felt that in being identified, his wife, Dr. Willa Brown, could be remembered for making one last contribution to the wellbeing of people struggling with serious illness.

Suzanne Holmes, Ed.D., for being an All-Weather Friend during the worst time of my life and for her encouragement and unfailing wisdom.

Craig Kayser, Editorial Director of Truewind Press, for his incisive criticism, expert advice, and sense of humor.

Andrea Doudera, Beverly Mills Gyllenhaal, Charlotte Goodman, Ph.D., Addison Hobbs, Ph.D., Elizabeth Meade Howard, Emily Long, Julie Matsumoto, M.D., Ellen Phipps, and Missie Rennie Taylor, all of whom offered critically important advice or served as readers.

I also thank close friends who read sections along the way, providing me with invaluable feedback. They allowed me to turn into a hibernating, self-absorbed, preoccupied person, as I wrangled through producing a book and establishing The All-Weather Friend as a new brand, without vanishing from my life forever. Specific among them is John Baker, who was subject to more of my handwringing than anyone else and bore it with great equanimity. Thanks to John, as well, for being a steady anchor when Bells, my beloved collie, died of cancer and through my own scare on that front. He has contributed to the book and to my life in more ways than I can mention.

I wish, particularly, to honor with the All-Weather Friend book series my late husband, Wayne S. Cail, M.D., through whom I learned the meaning of compassion and the power of friendship.

Finally, I acknowledge my brother and only sibling, Greg McDaniel, as a silent driving force behind the book. Greg was my "Irish twin" and best friend growing up. He spent his first real estate commission check on a pair of earrings for me many years ago. Greg died suddenly at the age of fifty, while raking leaves. I lovingly dedicate my book to him.

WORKS CONSULTED

Alzheimer, Alois. "About a Peculiar Disease of the Cerebral Cortex." *Psychiatrie und Psychisch-Gertichtliche Medizin* (1907). Translated by L. Jarvik and H. Greenson. *Alzheimer's Disease and Associated Disorders* 1, no. 1 (1987): 3–8.

Alzheimer's Association. "2012 Alzheimer's Disease Facts and Figures." *Alzheimer's and Dementia* 8, no. 2 (March 2012): 131–168.

———. "Risk factors for Alzheimer's disease." *Alzheimer's Association*. 2012, http://www.alz.org.

———. "Know the Ten Signs." *Alzheimer's Association*. 2012, http://www.alz. org.

The Alzheimer's Project. Produced by Sheila Nevins and Maria Shriver; Series Producer, John Hoffman. 2009. New York: HBO Documentary Films. DVD.

Ballard, Edna, Lisa P. Gwyther, and T. Patrick Toal. *Pressure Points: Alzheimer's and Anger.* Durham, N.C.: Duke University Press, 2000.

Belluck, Pam. "New Drug Trial Seeks to Stop Alzheimer's Before It Starts." *The New York Times.* 15 May 2012, http://nyti.ms/1eGIEDc.

Bird, T. D. et al. "Characteristics of Familial Alzheimer's Disease in Nine Kindreds of Volga German Ancestry." *Progress in Clinical Biological Research* 317 (1989): 229–234.

Brodaty, Henry and Marika Donkin. "Family Caregivers of People with Dementia." *Dialogues in Clinical Neuroscience* 11, no. 2 (June 2009): 217–228.

Brunnstrom, H. R. and E. M. Englund. "Cause of Death in Patients with Dementia Disorders [Abstract]." *European Journal of Neurology* 16, no. 4 (April 2009): 488–92.

Covey, Stephen. *The Seven Habits of Highly Effective People*. New York: The Free Press, 1989.

Daly, Jennette M. "Evidence-Based Practice Guideline: Elder Abuse Prevention." *Journal of Gerontological Nursing* 37, no. 11 (November 2011): 11–17.

Davidson, Ann. *Alzheimer's: A Love Story: One Year in My Husband's Journey.* Secaucus, N.J.: Carol Publishing Group, 1997.

DeKosky, Steven. "Pathology and Pathways of Alzheimer's Disease with an Update on New Developments in Treatment." *Journal of the American Geriatric Society* 51, no. 5 (2003): S314–20.

Doraiswamy, P. Murali, Lisa P Gwyther, and Tina Adler. *The Alzheimer's Action Plan: What You Need to Know—and What You Can Do—About Memory Problems, from Prevention to Early Intervention and Care.* New York: St. Martin's Griffin, 2009.

Dubois, Bruno et al. "Research Criteria for the Diagnosis of Alzheimer's Disease: Revising the NINCDS-ADRDA Criteria." *The Lancet Neurology* 6, no. 8 (2007): 734–746.

Eikelenboom, Piet et al. "Whether, When and How Chronic Inflammation Increases the Risk of Developing Late-Onset Alzheimer's Disease [Abstract]." *Alzheimer's Research and Therapy* 4, no. 15 (June 2012): http://alzres.com/content/4/3/15.

Esparza, Thomas J. et al. "Amyloid-Beta Oligomerization in Alzheimer Dementia Versus High Pathology Controls." *Annals of Neurology* (online version of record published before inclusion in an issue): http://bit.ly/15xBhHo.

"Family Caregiving Stress Filled and Isolating." *ScienceDaily.* 22 April 2010, www.sciencedaily.com./releases/2010/04/100422112641.htm.

Farran, Carol J. et al. "Caring for Self While Caring for Others: The Two-Track Life of Coping with Alzheimer's Disease." *Journal of Gerontological Nursing* 30, no. 5 (2004): 38–46.

Feinberg, Lynn et al. "Valuing the Invaluable: 2011 Update: The Growing Contributions and Costs of Family Caregiving." *AARP Public Policy Institute.* July 2011, http://www.aarp.org/relationships/caregiving/info-07-2011/valuing-the-invaluable.html.

Fetterman, Mindy. "Becoming 'Parent of Your Parent' an Emotionally Wrenching Process." *USA Today*, 25 June 2007, http://usat.ly/lcpl4L.

Foer, Joshua. "Remember This." *National Geographic* (November, 2007): 32-57.

Fuhs, Molly. "CAF's Dr. Tanzi on the Latest Alzheimer's Genes." *Cure Alzheimer's Fund*. 18 April 2011, www.curealzfund.org.

Geldmacher, David S. "Cost Effectiveness of Drug Therapies for the Treatment of Alzheimer's Disease: A Brief Review." *Neuropsychiatric Disease and Treatment* 4, no. 3 (2008): 549–555.

Goedert, Michel and Bernardino Ghetti. "Alois Alzheimer: His Life and Times." *Brain Pathology* 17 (2007): 57–62.

Goedert, Michel and Maria Grazia Spillantini. "A Century of Alzheimer's Disease." *Science* 314, no. 5800 (2006): 777–781.

Grady, Denise. "When Illness Makes a Spouse a Stranger." *The New York Times*. 5 May 2012, http://nyti.ms/KDpdpv.

Graeber, Manuel B. "No Man Alone: The Rediscovery of Alois Alzheimer's Original Cases." *Brain Pathology* 9, no. 2 (2006): 237–240.

Graeber, Manuel B. and Parviz Mehraein. "Reanalysis of the First Case of Alzheimer's Disease." *European Archives of Psychiatry and Clinical Neuroscience* 249, Supplement no. 3 (December 1999): S10–S13.

Graeber, Manuel et al. "Rediscovery of the Case Described by Alois Alzheimer in 1911: Historical, Histological and Molecular Genetic Analysis." *Neurogenetics* 1, no. 1 (1997): 73–80.

Hardy, John. "A Hundred Years of Alzheimer's Disease Research." *Neuron* 52, no. 1 (2006): 3–13.

Hollingworth, Paul et al. "Common Variants at ABCA7, MS4A6A/MS4A4E, EPHA 1, CD33 and CD2AP Are Associated with Late-Onset Alzheimer's Disease." *Nature Genetics* 43, no. 5 (May 2011): 429–435.

Humpel, Christian and Tanja Hochstrasser. "Cerebrospinal Fluid and Blood Biomarkers in Alzheimer's Disease." *World Journal of Psychiatry* 1, no. 1 (December 2011): 8–18.

Kelly, B. "Dr. William Saunders Hallaran and Psychiatric Practice in Nine-teenth-Century Ireland." *Irish Journal of Medical Science* 177, no. 1 (March 2008): 79–84.

Khachaturian, Zaven S. and Teresa S. Radebaugh, eds. *Alzheimer's Disease: Cause(s), Diagnosis, Treatment and Care.* New York: CRC Press, 1996.

Kolata, Gina. "For Alzheimer's, Detection Advances Outpace Treatment Options." *The New York Times.* 15 November 2012, http://nyti.ms/1bmSRRQ.

———. "Rules Seek to Expand Diagnosis of Alzheimer's." *The New York Times.* 30 July 2010, http://nyti.ms/bx52NU.

Lanctot, Krista L., Ryan D. Rajaram, and Nathan Herrman. "Review: Therapy for Alzheimer's Disease: How Effective Are Current Treatments?" *Therapeutic Advances in Neurological Disorders* 2, no.3 (2009): 163–80.

Mace, Nancy L. and Peter V. Rabbins. *The 36-Hour Day: A Family Guide to Caring for People Who Have Alzheimer's Disease, Related Dementias, and Memory Loss.* Baltimore, Md.: The Johns Hopkins University Press, 2011.

Maurer, Konrad and Ulrike Maurer. *Alzheimer: The Life of a Physician and the Career of a Disease.* Translated by Neil Levi and Alastair Burns. New York: Columbia University Press, 2003.

Maurer, Konrad, Stephan Wolk, and Hector Gerbaldo. "Auguste D and Alzheimer's Disease." *The Lancet* 349, no. 9064 (May 1997): 1546–1549.

Mayeux, Richard. "Early Alzheimer's Disease." *New England Journal of Medicine* 362, no. 4 (10 June 2010): 2194–2201.

McCurry, Susan et al. "Insomnia in Caregivers of Persons with Dementia: Who is at Risk and What Can Be Done About It? [Abstract]" *Sleep Medicine Clinics* 4, no. 4 (December 2009): 519–526.

McIntyre, Maura and Ardra Cole. "Love Stories About Caregiving and Alzheimer's Disease." *Journal of Health Psychology* 13, no. 2 (2008): 213–225.

McKhann, Guy et al. "The Diagnosis of Alzheimer's Disease: Recommendations from the National Institute on Aging—Alzheimer's Association Workgroups on Diagnostic Guidelines for Alzheimer's Disease." *Alzheimer's and Dementia* 7, no. 3 (May 2011): 263–269.

McKhann, Guy et al., "Clinical Diagnosis of Alzheimer's Disease: Report of the NINCDS-ADRDA Work Groups Under Auspices of Department of Health and Human Services Task Force on Alzheimer's Disease." *Neurology* 34, no. 7 (1984): 939–944.

Mohamed, Somaia, Robert Rosenheck, and Lon Schreider. "Clinical Correlates of Caregiver Burden in Alzheimer's Disease." *Alzheimer's and Dementia* 5, no. 4 (July 2009): 228.

Mormino, E., J. et al. "Episodic Memory Loss Is Related to Hippocampal-Mediated-ß Amyloid Deposition in Elderly Subjects." *Brain* 132, no. 5 (2009): 1310–1323.

Morris, John C. "John Morris on Detecting Alzheimer's at the Preclinical Stage: Special Topic of Alzheimer's Disease Interview." *Science Watch,* October 2011, http://bit.ly/1aNKWhc.

Morris, John C. et al. "Pittsburgh Compound B Imaging and Prediction of Progression from Cognitive Normality to Symptomatic Alzheimer Disease." *Archives of Neurology* 66, no. 12 (2009): 1469–1475.

Nag, Adam C. et al. "Common Variants in MS4A4/MS4A6E, CD2uAP, CD33, and EPHA1 Are Associated with Late-Onset Alzheimer's Disease." *Nature Genetics* 43, no. 5 (May 2011): 436–441.

Peterson, Betsy. *Voices of Alzheimer's: Courage, Hope, and Love in the Face of Dementia.* Cambridge, Mass.: DaCapo Life Long, 2004.

Reisberg, Barry et al. "Outcome Over Seven Years of Healthy Adults With and Without Subjective Cognitive Impairment." *Alzheimer's and Dementia* 6, no. 1 (2010): 11–24.

Reisberg, Barry et al. "Evidence and Mechanisms of Retrogenesis in Alzheimer's Disease and Other Dementias." *American Journal of Alzheimer's and Other Dementias* 17, no 4 (July/August 2002): 202–212.

Right at Home. "Home Safety Checklist for Alzheimer's Caregivers." *Caring Right at Home.* September 2007, http://bit.ly/196UVZp.

Rockoff, Jonathan D. "New Data Released on Lilly Alzheimer's Drug." *The Wall Street Journal,* 9 October 2012, B4.

Rosa, E. et al., "Needs of Caregivers of Patients with Dementia." *Archives of Gerontology and Geriatrics* 51, no. 1 (July 2010): 54–58.

Scoville, William Beecher and Brenda Milner. "Classic Articles: Loss of Recent Memory After Bilateral Hippocampal Lesions." *Journal of Neuropsychiatry and Clinical Neurosciences* 12 (February 2000): 103–113.

Serrano-Pozo, Alberto et al. "Neuropathogical Alterations in Alzheimer Disease." *Cold Spring Harbor Perspectives in Medicine* 1, no. 1 (September 2011): http://www.perspectivesinmedicine.org/content/1/1/a006189. abstract.

Shaffer, Jennifer L. et al. "Predicting Cognitive Decline in Subjects at Risk for Alzheimer's Disease by Using Combined Cerebrospinal Fluid, MR Imaging, and PET Biomarkers." *Radiology* (Published online before print December 11, 2012): http://www.ncbi.nlm.nih.gov/pubmed/23232293.

Shriver, Maria. *Alzheimer's In America: The Shriver Report on Women and Alzheimer's.* New York: Free Press, 2011.

Simmons, B. Brent and Brett Hartmann. "Evaluation of Suspected Dementia." *American Family Physician* 84, no. 8 (October 15, 2011): 895–902.

Small, Gary and Gigi Vorgan. *The Alzheimer's Prevention Program: Keep Your Brain Healthy for the Rest of Your Life.* New York: Workman Publishing Company, 2012.

Strait, Julia Evangelou. "Clue to Alzheimer's Cause Found in Brain Samples." *Washington State University in St. Louis Newsroom.* 22 October 2012, http://news.wustl.edu/news/Pages/24431.aspx).

Strauch, Carl F. "The Date of Emerson's *Terminus*." *PMLA* 65, no. 4 (1950): 360.

Strobel, Gabrielle G. "Alzheimer Research Forum Report: Tübingen: The Man Behind the Eponym." *Journal of Alzheimer's Disease* 11, no. 1 (2007):131–133.

Swyers, Jim. "Peculiar material disbanding unruly mobs of proteins." *Pittmed* (Spring 2007): 23–27.

University of Florida. "Ways to Help Communication—Tip Sheet." *University of Florida Center for Research on Telehealth and Assistive Technology.* 28 August 2007, www.alzonline.phhp.ufl.edu/en/reading/communication.php.

Weimer, David and Mark A. Sager. "Early Identification and Treatment of Alzheimer's Disease: Social and Fiscal Outcomes." *Alzheimer's and Dementia* 5, no. 3 (May 2009): 215–226.

Windholtz, George. "Psychiatric Treatment and the Condition of the Mentally Disturbed at Berlin's Carite in the Early Decades of the Nineteenth Century." *History of Psychiatry* 6, no. 22 (1995): 136–157.

Wippold, Franz, N. Cairns, David Holtzman, and John C. Morris. "Neuropathology for the Neuroradiologist: Plaques and Tangles." *American Journal of Neuroradiology* 29 (January 2008): 18–22.

Wolpe, David. *Making Loss Matter: Creating Meaning in Difficult Times.* New York: Riverhead Books, 1999.

Wright, Joan F., Mary E. Doherty, and Linda G. Dumas. "Caregiver Burden: Three Voices—Three Realities." *Nursing Clinics of North America* 44, no. 2 (June 2009): 209–221.

Zilka, Norbert and Michael Novak. "The Tangled Story of Alois Alzheimer." *Bratisl Lek Listy* 107, no. 9–10 (2006): 343–345.

INDEX

TOPICS AND QUESTIONS FOR DISCUSSION

1. Have you faced a difficult experience when your friends didn't know how to help or what to say?

2. Have you ever been unable to understand what a friend was going through because you had not shared a similar experience? How did you handle it?

3. Are we ready as a culture to hear a message of inclusivity and friendship for people with dementia or are we too afraid of the condition?

4. In the early-stage story (pp. 19–27), Adelle's husband gives a "dramatic example of love and humanity" (p. 24). What do you think makes a person able to put aside his or her needs and frustrations and go the distance as a caregiver, often for a period of many years?

5. Chapter 2 begins with a list of things not to say to someone in early-stage Alzheimer's disease. Do you agree with this list, and can you add any items to it?

6. Are there strategies in chapters 2 and 3 that apply to all of our close relationships, not just friendships with Alzheimer's patients and caregivers?

7. Based on your experience, which of the strategies in these chapters are the most important to remember and put into practice?

8. Cathryn (chapter 4) is unable to cope with Neal due to her health and his physical size, personality changes, and level of decline. The chapter opens with a quote from Cathryn: "We all agree in support group that the marriage ends" (p. 59). Is this true? What are the differences between marriage and friendship that might allow friendship to survive dementia, if marriage cannot?

9. The author recommends that we accept what a person in mid-stage says and perceives without correcting facts or arguing. How hard is this to do? What makes it hard?

10. Chapter 5 provides a communication toolkit for helping a friend with mid-stage Alzheimer's. How must we redefine our concept of friendship to allow for the relational problems AD causes?

11. Consider the strategies in chapter 6 for helping a mid-stage caregiver. Are each of these strategies relevant in friendships, no matter what the circumstances? Can you think of an example of when a friend gave you advice you didn't want to hear, or inadvertently made a difficult situation worse by being insensitive? Have you been guilty of this yourself?

12. Velma's story (chapter 7) isn't altogether negative and sad. What makes it bittersweet?

13. Consider this quote from chapter 8: "A disease can change the way the future will play out. It cannot change the past" (p. 104), encouraging us not to lose track of the things we've loved about a person all along. What are some ways we can keep a friend or loved one's dementia from overriding our own good memories?

14. The subtitle of one of the strategies for helping a late-stage caregiver is *Tend to the Tears* (p.113). Why are we so uncomfortable when a person cries, or are we?

15. The author briefly discusses her conception of grief (pp. 117–18). What do you think of the analogy she uses to describe grief? When you've grieved, what helped you feel better? How long did grief go on for you?

16. Bert says his love for his wife "continues but with a changed circumstance" (p. 128). Can friendship with a person suffering from dementia continue but with a changed circumstance?

17. Page 136 has a tongue-in-cheek, how-not-to-write-it letter the author confesses was based on one she actually received from a friend. Have you had an experience in which a friend made an unhappy circumstance in your life seem even worse by bragging?

18. Which of the suggestions in chapter 11, *Seven Ways to Stay Connected*, would be the easiest for you to do as a friend or to accept as a caregiver?

19. In chapter 12, *The Dinner Party*, the author hosts a party attended by a woman, Elaine, then in mid-to-late stage AD, and her caregiving husband. Several of the people she invited, she says, declined when they realized Elaine would be among the guests. Why do we have such a difficult time accepting other people's challenges or differences and responding compassionately?

20. This book was written for friends, from the perspective of a friend. The strategies and suggestions are meant to be relatively easy and realistic for a busy friend with limited time. The author does not include helping with the more intimate, difficult acts of caregiving for this reason. The book is not meant to portray how terrible Alzheimer's disease can be under certain circumstances but rather to encourage people not to abandon (in fear or awkwardness) the friends and loved ones who struggle with it. Do you think she accomplished her purpose—to create a guide for the All-Weather Friend? Why or why not?

21. In the epilogue, the author relates a true story about a man who demonstrated an inexplicable understanding of an event he could not possibly have witnessed. The brain has been described by other writers as the transmitter ("the television set") of a greater consciousness which remains intact—but can no longer be perceived, due to the broken transmitter or failed mind. What do you think of this idea?

22. Do you think people fear that Alzheimer's disease is contagious (see note 31, p. 177)? Is this fear rational?

23. What does *Terminus* by Ralph Waldo Emerson (p. 201–02) say about how Emerson regarded his worsening dementia? What lessons can we find in the poem?

24. Do you have a true All-Weather Friend in your life? How rare is this kind of friend in the present day and age, in which self-sufficiency and busyness are prized, and social media has become a main way connecting?

Terminus

It is time to be old,
To take in sail:
The god of bounds,
Who sets to seas a shore,
Come to me in his final rounds,
And said: "No more!
No farther shoot
Thy broad ambitious branches, and thy root.
Fancy departs; no more invent;
Contract thy firmament
To compass of tent.
There's not enough for this and that,
Make thy option which of two;
Economize the failing river,
Not the less revere the Giver,
Leave the many and hold the few.
Timely wise accept the terms,
Soften the fall with wary foot;
A little while
Still plan and smile,
And, fault of novel germs,
Mature the unfallen fruit.
Curse, if thou wilt, thy sires,
Bad husbands of their fires,

Who, when they gave thee breath,
Failed to bequeath
The needful sinew stark as once,
The Baresark marrow to thy bones,
But left a legacy of ebbing veins,
Inconstant heat and nerveless reins,
Amid the Muses, left thee deaf and dumb,
Amid the gladiators, halt and numb."

As the bird trims her to the gale,
I trim myself to the storm of time,
I man the rudder, reef the sail,
Obey the voice at eve obeyed at prime:
"Lowly faithful, banish fear,
Right onward drive unharmed;
The port, well worth the cruise, is near,
And every wave is charmed."

— RALPH WALDO EMERSON,
written about 1866, as his mind began to fail

Mary Cail, Ph.D. became an advocate for Alzheimer's patients and their caregivers after the tragic death of her husband, when she began working with the elderly and with the Alzheimer's Association as a way of finding comfort for herself. The idea of The All-Weather Friend and this book evolved out of her experience. Mary leads patient and caregiver support groups for the Alzheimer's Association of Central and Western Virginia. She received 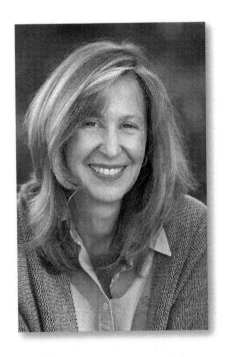 her doctoral degree in Counselor Education and Supervision from the University of Virginia. Her work has been covered in *The Miami Herald, The Seattle Times, The Washington Post*, and many other publications. Visit her website: www.allweatherfriend.com.

Made in the USA
Lexington, KY
20 January 2017